UNDERSTAND PH
REGAIN YOUR HEALTH
LOSE WEIGHT

ALKALINE DIET

COOKBOOK

BY MELISSA BENNETT

Table of Contents

Chapter Five: Salad Alkaline Diet Recipes   86

Chapter Six: Snacks Alkaline Diet Recipes   96

Chapter Seven: Deserts Alkaline Diet Recipes   108

Conclusion   121

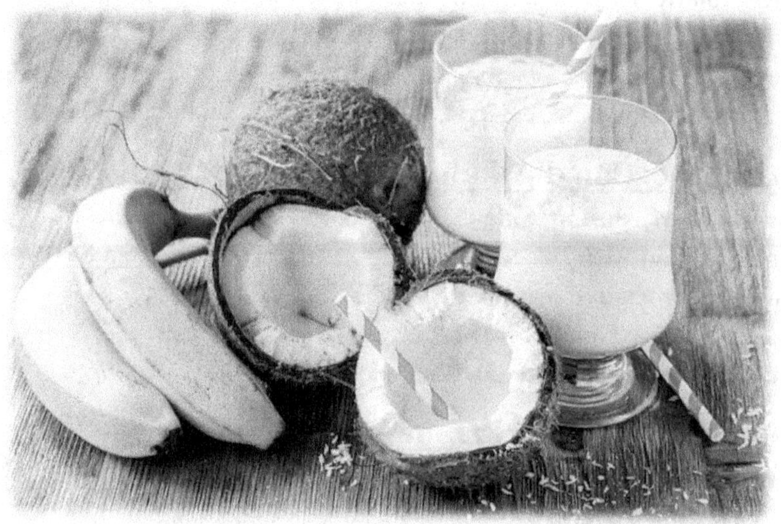

Introduction

You are what you eat!

This saying could not be any closer to the truth. Everything that we ingest contributes to the way we live and the way our bodies function. If we live off highly processed, unhealthy food on a regular basis, our bodies will become subject to a number of health complications – hypertension, coronary heart disease, Type 2 Diabetes, etc. We don't think about our food choices until it's too late.

Many people tend to spend the majority of their youth eating unhealthy foods until it is too late. By the time they start making healthier food choices, it's too late. The damage has already been done. Any healthy eating done afterwards won't be as effective. Prevention is always better than cure.
This applies to the way we treat our bodies. We shouldn't wait for something within us to be broken before we try to fix it. We should treat our bodies the same way we treat our prized possessions – with care and careful consideration. The foods we consume have a great impact on our bodies.

As mentioned earlier, if we try to fill our bodies with food that has little or no nutritional value, our bodies will suffer. If more people were to pay greater attention to how they treat their bodies, many health complications would be at an all-time low.

A few signs that you have too much acid in your body:

Sluggishness

Sluggishness occurs when someone is always tired, unable to remain alert, and struggles to feel rested – even after a full night's rest. If you feel sluggish on a regular basis then this is a clear indicator that something is wrong. We are not designed to be tired all the time. The purpose of sleep is to give us the rest and energy we need in order to move forward with the next day.

If that isn't happening the way it should, then it is clear that there is an imbalance in your system. Most people make the mistake of combating these feelings of sluggishness with highly caffeinated beverages – and lots of sugar. Both of these things are known to make the body feel worse. Instead of helping your body, you are actually harming it by feeding it so many toxins.

A build-up of acid will do this to your body. It will rob you of your energy and have you in a constant state of fatigue and sluggishness. If you try to remedy your fatigue with coffee, soda, and other toxic beverages, you will also mess up your sleep cycle – which will worsen the situation even more. These drinks are not designed to help you. They are designed to give you a quick buzz that will come with a number of toxic repercussions. It makes it almost impossible for you to wake up with the energy you need to tackle the day. Most of these stimulants are acidic and leave you feeling worse than you were before.

Oral Signs

When acid builds up in the body, it can have a serious effect on the mouth. One of the signs of this will be in your saliva. A sticky, dry feeling in your mouth; constantly feeling thirsty; and even a dry feeling in your throat are signs of your saliva being overly acidic.

Other known signs are a burning or tingling sensation in your mouth – particularly on the tongue – as well as problems speaking, tasting, chewing or swallowing food. If the situation persists, mouth ulcers will start to develop.

Your teeth will become affected after a while as well – often becoming sensitive and gradually corroded. In extreme cases, the gums become inflamed and the teeth become loose within their sockets. This will lead to worse complications if care is not taken.

Eye Signs

If you have too much acid in your body, you may also find signs of it in your eyes. If your eyes tear up very easily or appear to be very irritated, do not take this lightly. If left unattended, your corneas and eyelids could become inflamed too – leading to bouts of conjunctivitis.

Conjunctivitis is also known as "pinkeye". It occurs when the conjunctiva – the mucous membrane that covers the front of the eye – becomes inflamed. These are some of the symptoms of conjunctivitis:

- Increased amount of tears
- Itchy or burning eyes
- Blurred vision
- Thick, yellowish discharge that crusts over the eyelashes – particularly after sleep
- Discharge from the eye that is white or green in color
- Increased light sensitivity

Signs in the Digestive Tract

Acidity tends to display itself intensely in the digestive tract. If you have too much acid in your body, you will end up regurgitating it or suffering from acid reflux. Acid reflux is often characterized by a burning chest pain known as heartburn. Discomfort and pain can range from minimal to extreme. Another sign of acid reflux is regurgitating sour acid back up into your throat or your mouth.

Other symptoms of acid reflux are:

- Bloating
- Frequent burping
- Incessant hiccups
- Unexplained weight loss
- A chronic sore throat
- Stomach ulcers and gastritis are also capable of developing as a result of too much acid being in your body.

Gastritis occurs when the stomach lining becomes inflamed. Symptoms of the condition are constant abdominal pain, unwavering nausea, vomiting, and, in some instances, appetite loss, bloating and indigestion.

Emotional and Mental Signs

Having an acidic body can also lead to your mental and emotional state being negatively affected. Loss of motivation and decreased interest in activities you once loved are a couple of the symptoms that could occur due to high body acid content. If you have an acid problem, you may find yourself feeling nervous, irritable, and very sensitive to loud noises. You will also become more likely to become depressed.

High body acid content is a result of the foods one consumes. People may not realize it but many of the foods they assume are "normal" are actually contributing to the discomfort and health complications they experience on a regular basis.

The alkaline diet is a specialized diet that aims to assist people with losing weight, maintain a healthy bodily system, and live longer, fulfilling lives.

Chapter One: What is the Alkaline Diet?

The alkaline diet is also known as the alkaline ash diet or the acid-alkaline diet. The purpose of the alkaline diet is to assist with balancing the pH level of the fluids in your body – including your blood and your urine.

The alkaline diet encourages the consumption of foods that are said to influence an acid-base homeostasis in the body. Acid-base homeostasis is essential for regular body function, cell metabolism, and the overall physiological state. The importance of this regulation is evident in a variety of physiologic malfunctions that occur when the body's pH is either too high or too low.

The kidneys play a major role in regulating the metabolic component of the body by balancing the concentration of acid-base foods ingested. In Essence the kidneys have to reabsorb all the filtered bicarbonate in the process of creating new bicarbonate to replenish compounds that were ingested by acids (normal or pathologic). The process of producing or generating new bicarbonate is done through net acid excretion. Net acid excretion is the net amount of acid that is released (or excreted) in urine per unit per time.

Under regular conditions, one third to one half of the net acid excretion from the kidneys is in the form of acids that are known as titratable. Titratable acids play an important role in renal (kidney) function. The rest of the one half or two thirds, under regular conditions, is excreted in the form of ammonium. Ammonium is acidic. When acid-base homeostasis is not occurring, health complications can occur. In clinical medicine, most complications can be traced back to systems that are involved with acid-base transportation in the kidneys.

The alkaline diet is based on the belief that the foods you consume can alter the acidity or the alkalinity of your body. This acidity-alkalinity relation is known as the pH value of your body and will be discussed in forthcoming paragraphs.

Basically, this is how it works:

When you consume food, your body takes it in and metabolizes it. While your food is being metabolized by your body, energy is being extracted from it – this energy is known as calories. This process can be viewed as a burning process. Your body is burning the food you consume in order to give your body the energy it requires. This process happens in a slow, gradual, and controlled manner. As your food burns, an ash residue is left behind. Think of the grey or white ash that is left behind when wood is burnt in a furnace. That is the kind of ash that forms in your body – except it comes from food, not wood.

This ash can be acidic, alkaline, or neutral. Components of the alkaline diet state that this ash can directly impact the acidity of your body. If you eat foods that produce predominantly acidic ash, your body will become acidic. If you eat foods that produce alkaline ash, your body will become alkaline. Neutral ash has no effect – but such ash is rarely produced.

Acidic ash is responsible for making you susceptible to illness and chronic disease, but alkaline ash is considered to be protective. The purpose of the alkaline diet is to protect your body from becoming overly acidic. In the previous section, I highlighted some of the detrimental symptoms of having too much acid in your body.

Having a high acidic content in your body can leave you vulnerable to many unpleasant diseases. Unfortunately, the problem with the standard diet is that it promotes the consumption of acidic foods.

Researchers believe that when it comes to the total acid content of the typical human diet, there have been significant changes from what was eaten during the hunter gatherer times and what is eaten now. Advancements within agriculture and general industrialization have led to increased sodium in our foods and less potassium, chloride and magnesium.

As mentioned earlier, our kidneys play a role in maintaining the levels of our electrolytes – calcium, potassium, chloride, and magnesium. When our bodies become overly exposed to acidic substances, electrolytes will target and fight the acidity. If they are not compensated for, an imbalance will occur in the body.

The sodium content in most people's bodies is far more than the potassium content – this is a result of the changes in our diet over the years. Many people – adults and children – are on high-sodium diets that are not supplying them with sufficient amounts of potassium, magnesium and antioxidants – as well as important vitamins and other fiber. The standard Western diet is rich in processed fats, simple sugars, and salt (which contains sodium and chloride).

Many people are walking around with high acidic contents in their bodies, thus weakening their immune systems and making them susceptible to many diseases. Within the last couple of decades, we have seen cases of heart disease, cancer, and other terrible diseases rise. The foods we eat play a major role in this rise. Some people have tried to counter this claim, but it is true.

The quality of our foods is affecting our bodily health. This is why people are ageing faster, losing organ function, and experiencing tissue and bone mass degeneration. Acid is robbing people of their youth and their lives. This is why the alkaline diet is important. It was formulated to reverse the damage done in order to restore good health to everyone.

The diet promotes the consumption of healthier, wholesome foods – which will be discussed further – over less beneficial foods (mainly processed and refined foods that are high in sugar, sodium, and saturated fats). This really is a matter of life or death. The fact that you are reading this book means you are headed in the right direction.

Why is the Alkaline Diet Helpful?

A Healthier Body

Following a healthy diet is a sure way to keep your body in top condition. When your diet consists of you eating the right foods – in the right quantities – your whole body will benefit from it. A healthy diet can keep your bones and teeth strong. Your bones and your teeth need a mineral known as calcium in order to remain strong. When you consume healthy doses of calcium (often found in fish, dark green vegetables, soya products, fresh fruit juices, etc.) your bones and your teeth receive the fortification that they need. A calcium-rich diet will also prevent osteoporosis (bone loss) as you get older.

A healthy diet also keeps your heart healthy – which is of the utmost importance. A body cannot function effectively if the heart is not healthy. A diet that consists of fruits, vegetables, and other healthy foods will help keep your heart in the best condition possible. Too much salt and saturated fats can lead to heart complications and heart-related diseases. This is why people turn to dieting – to regulate their salt and fat intake in order to prevent such from happening.

Your body will also be supplied with an ample amount of energy when you live on a healthy, balanced diet. Most people live demanding lives that require them to be active for more than twelve to fifteen hours a day. A healthy diet is the only way that one will be able to attain the energy needed for such demanding days. Nutrients from the foods you eat will also assist with growth, muscle repair, and staying immune to various diseases.

Disease Prevention

As one becomes older, they become more prone to health complications and diseases that could affect them for the rest of their lives. Diabetes (type 2) is one of such disease. This is a lifelong condition that can cause a person's blood sugar levels to become dangerously high. In the case of type 2 Diabetes, the body is unable to produce sufficient insulin to control the blood sugar levels. If left untreated, a person will die. A healthy, balanced diet will help you keep your saturated fat intake at an acceptable level, while ensuring that you consume enough whole grains to reduce the risk of developing this disease.

A healthy, balanced diet will also keep you from developing heart-related diseases, hypertension, and high cholesterol levels. The risk of developing these diseases also increase with one's age. If healthy eating choices are not made, one could end up having their life cut short by one of these diseases. The same way saturated fats, processed sugar, and a high salt intake can lead to type 2 diabetes, is the same way these factors can lead to a number of other diseases.

Prevention is always better than attempting to cure a disease. The best way to prevent these diseases from occurring is ensuring that your diet is healthy and balanced. Foods such as fish – trout and salmon can help lower your risk of developing heart disease. These fish are known to contain high levels of the omega-3 fatty acids – which are very good for the heart's health.

Weight Control

Weight loss/regulation is one of the main reasons why people choose to incorporate healthy diets into their life. Obesity has become a global problem, with WHO recording that, as of 2016, more than 1.9 billion adults aged 18 and older were considered to be overweight. Obesity is majorly a result of poor food choices. Many people are not eating the foods that they should be eating.

This is due to laziness, little time to prepare meals, apathy, health-related issues, and a number of other reasons. It does not help that many popular food corporations are known for producing foods that have little to no nutritional value. Obesity is no longer just an adult problem. The same WHO report stated that 41 million children across the world were said to be overweight or obese in 2016. Parents are not giving their children the right foods to eat and it is leading to a global crisis.

A healthy, balanced diet is one of the main ways to get rid of unwanted pounds and regulate a healthy body weight. Exercise is often spoken of as the main way for one to lose weight, but without a healthy diet all exercise will go to waste. There is a popular saying that states that weight loss/muscle gain is 25% gym (exercise) and 75% diet. It is clear that if one desires to attain or maintain a healthy weight, they need to make sure that their food choices are healthy, balanced and beneficial for their bodies.

The problem many people face, when it comes to dieting, is actually finding the right diet. It is very hard to find a long-term, reliable diet. Most diets that are formulated today are created by people who are looking to make money off of people. I won't name any but I am sure that a few names have already popped into your mind. The weight loss may come rapidly but it will not stay. Weight loss should be a by-product of exercise and a healthy diet. If anyone tries to tell you otherwise, do not listen to them.

The alkaline diet is that healthy diet that can give you the healthy body you need, while regulating your weight loss, and warding off disease. It was designed with the intention of providing overall bodily health. The alkaline diet can also slow the ageing process, prevent arthritis and diabetes, and have you feeling great on a regular basis.

Your energy levels will be boosted, along with your memory, and headaches, bloating and muscle pain are things you will not have to worry about again. All these benefits simply coming from increasing your intake of alkaline foods, while decreasing the amount of acidic foods you consume. It really is that simple! Once you get the hang of it, you will be very glad.

What is Ph, Acidic Food and Alkaline Food?

Ph

The mistake scores of people tend to make is that they hardly ever think about the balance between acid and alkaline in blood. This balance – between acid and alkaline - is also known as the body's pH level. A stable level is key for a person to be healthy. In earlier segments of this chapter, we went through the various complications that occur because of a present imbalance in a person's body. A balanced pH will enable our bodies to remain protected from the inside out. Diseases and any other health disorders will struggle to affect a body with a balanced ph.

When an imbalance occurs in the body, it will allow unhealthy organisms to enter the body's system and compromise it. This results in damaged tissues and major organs – which leads to an immune system that is at risk.

The term "pH" is actually the shortened term for "potential of hydrogen". This is the measure of the presence of acid and alkaline in a solution. This is also measured from a scale of 0 to 14. When a solution is highly acidic, the pH value will be low. When the solution is more alkaline, the pH value will be much higher. When a solution is a pH of 7 it means that it is perfectly neutral. The healthiest – and most recommended – pH is one that is slightly alkaline. Numerically, one would want to achieve a pH of 7.365. This number will definitely fluctuate as the day goes by but the normal range should be between 6 and 7.5.

These are the factors that cause acidity in the body:

- The use of narcotics and alcohol
- Overusing antibiotics and over-the-counter drugs
- The overindulgence of artificially sweetened products
- Declining level of nutrients in foods.
- Dangerously low levels of fiber in a person's typical diet
- A lack of proper exercise
- Eating too much animal meat – especially when they are fed from non-grass sources

If you've been experiencing any symptoms that could point to a presence of high levels of acid in your body, then take a look at the above list and determine whether any of these factors are contributing to your present condition.

Acid-forming Foods

- Cold cut meats – ham, turkey, etc.
- Eggs
- Lentils
- Oats
- Corn flakes
- Traditional meats – beef, pork, and chicken
- Milk
- Peanuts and walnuts
- Rice
- White bread

It is advisable to keep in mind that while some of these foods, like eggs and various nuts and grains, may be acidic in your body, you should not let this stop you from eating them. They still contain a great deal of health benefits, such as omega-3 fatty acids and necessary antioxidants, which your body needs in order to function properly. The best way to gain and maintain a healthy balance in your body is in the word "balance" itself. Balance between foods that are acidic and foods that are alkaline must be reached in order for your body to reach the perfect pH balance. It is possible for the body to become too alkaline – which is counter-productive. It is all about balance.

This diet does not encourage you to eat foods that are processed - such as canned and packaged products, convenience foods, etc. These foods are considered too acidic and they will have a negative impact on your body. Taking in alcohol and caffeinated drinks is not advisable either. These substances will negatively affect your body's health, which is not the goal here.

 You should know that this diet will involve abstaining from many foods. Some people consider the diet to be challenging because of this very factor. But if you are serious about improving your body's health, then these changes will be worthwhile. The initial months, after starting the diet, may be challenging, but once you get the hang of it, you will be grateful that you decided to eliminate most of these unhealthy and non-beneficial foods from your diet.

Alkaline foods

These are more of the foods you will be consuming during this diet. Most recommended foods for this diet are mushrooms, fruits and vegetables – preferably fresh. These foods contain great levels of nutrients that will leave your body feeling healthier, lighter, and stronger. Foods like citrus, dates, and even spinach will be the types of foods you will be eating on a regular basis.

Funny enough, foods that are thought to be acidic – e.g. grapefruits – are not unhealthy for the body. They actually contribute to the alkalinity of the body. They end up providing a totally opposite effect as well.

Raw foods – uncooked fruits and vegetables – are known to have a life-boosting effect on your body and the way it functions. It is believed that cooking foods decreases the essential minerals in these foods. This diet will encourage you to increase your intake of raw foods so that you can get all the nutritional goodness that you need. The best way to take these foods, without losing the nutrients, is through juicing them or partially steaming them. Try not to boil or fry these foods – they will have no nutritional value.

Another key aspect of this diet is alkaline water. This water has an alkaline pH that will greatly benefit your body. If you are unable to locate this type of water, you can opt for distilled water too. These options are way better than water that comes from the tap or plastic bottles. Adding ingredients like lemon, baking soda, or pH drops to your water will also boost its alkalinity.

Raw, green beverages will also form a common part of your diet. They are made from grasses and green vegetables (that can also come in powdered form). They are full of foods formed from alkaline and chlorophyll – which alkalizes the blood.

How to follow (what to eat, what to avoid, how to effectively balance acid foods with alkaline foods)

You need to put a great deal of effort into making sure that the foods you purchase for your diet are organic. Experts have noted that an important consideration, when it comes to this particular diet, is for the dieter to become conscious of the quality of the soil his or her fruits and vegetables were grown in.

Fruits and vegetables that are grown in soil that is totally organic, the kind of soil that happens to be dense with minerals, will have more beneficial properties for the diet, compared to produce grown in inorganic soil. Research has also shown that the quality of fruits and vegetables can be directly affected by the condition of the soil they are grown in – mainly, their vitamin and mineral content. This shows that not all foods that are deemed alkaline possess the same nutritional benefits.

The recommended pH for organic soil, in order for the production of nutritiously abundant fruits and beneficial vegetables, is found within the range of six and seven. Acidic soil with a pH below 6 will greatly reduce the amount of calcium and magnesium in the produce. Soil with a pH above 7 will result in iron, manganese, copper and zinc that is chemically unavailable. But soil that taken care of with organic materials – fertilizer and other chemicals - is the healthiest soil that should be used for the growth of top quality vegetables and fruits.

If you would like to know what your body's pH level is before you go on this diet, you can test it with strips that can be bought from a pharmacy close to you. To test the level, you can use your urine or saliva – the choice is yours.

If you opt for the urine option, you should use your second batch of urine of the day (preferably from the morning) because it will provide you with the best results. A chart should come with the testing kit, and it will help you understand all the information you need to know about your pH level and the way forward. If you choose to test your level during the day, the best time to do so would be an hour before – or two hours after – a meal. If you test your pH with your saliva, the best pH range to stay in is between 6.8 and 7.2.

Ideal Foods to Consume During This Diet:

As mentioned earlier on in the book, fresh fruits and vegetables are among the foods that will benefit your body the most during the alkaline diet. These are the fruits and vegetables you should incorporate in your meals:

- Mushrooms
- Citrus fruits
- Dates and raisins
- Spinach and kale
- Grapefruit
- Avocado
- Tomatoes
- Alfalfa grass
- Cucumber
- Wheat grass
- Garlic

- Ginger
- Cabbage
- Celery
- Watermelon
- Ripe bananas

You need to try and ensure that the majority of the foods you eat – **fruits and vegetables** – are uncooked. **Raw fruits and vegetables** are known to consist of life-giving properties that cooked produce cannot give you. Cooked food causes alkalizing minerals to deplete. By increasing the amount of raw foods, you eat, through juicing, partially steaming, or just eating your fruits and vegetables as they are, you are allowing your body to ingest the alkaline properties that need to be ingested.

Plant proteins are also a major necessity – almonds, butter beans (almost all beans are very good choices).

Alkaline water: This water consists of a 9-11. If you cannot access alkaline water, a good alternative is distilled water. I also recommend that you consume water that has been filtered from a reverse osmosis filter – it may be a little acidic in nature but it is much better than water that comes from the taps – or even bottled water. Another way to boost the alkalinity of your water is by adding pH drops, lemon, lime or baking soda.

You'll also have to incorporate **green beverages** into the foods you consume as well. There are important nutrients that you need to garner from them. As mentioned in the previous section, most green vegetables and grasses that are used for green drinks contain chlorophyll – which is very efficient when it comes to alkalizing the blood.

Foods to Avoid:

The consumption of acidic food should be kept to a minimum. If you eat too many acidic foods, your body's pH balance will be affected and your attempt at trying the alkaline diet will be for nothing. Foods that are capable of increasing the acidity in your body are:

- Foods that contain high levels of sodium content – processed foods are known to consist of high amounts of table salt – which can also go by the name sodium chloride. Sodium chloride can be responsible for constricting blood vessels and also creating a greater presence of acidity in the body.
- Traditional forms of meats (poultry, red meat, etc.) and refrigerated cuts (ham, salami, etc.)
- All processed cereals (e.g. corn flakes)
- All types of eggs
- Drinks that are caffeinated or contain considerable amounts of alcohol
- All forms of whole wheat foods – oats, all types of grains, whether they are whole or not, contribute to the presence of acid in your body. Processed corn or wheat tend to be the main culprits, if you are on a traditional American diet.
- Milk – one of the major causes of osteoporosis can be traced back to the consumption of dairy products that are high in calcium. This is because they are known to create the presence of acidity in the body. When the bloodstream contains high levels of acid, it will access the calcium in the bones and take it (due to its alkaline properties) in order to balance the pH level in the body. The best way to prevent osteoporosis from occurring is by eating a lot of vegetables that are leafy, green, and alkaline.
- Peanuts, walnuts and other types of nuts
- All packaged grain products such as pasta, white and brown rice, as well as white and brown bread.

Foods are not the only things that can contribute to the high acidity in your body. There are habits and other external factors that can contribute to your body's acidity too. The major offenders include:

- Substance abuse – alcohol, narcotics, etc.
- High caffeine intake
- Overusing antibiotics
- Artificial sweeteners
- Prolonged stress
- Low levels of fiber in one's regular diet
- Lack of exercise
- An excess of animal meat in one's diet – especially when the meat is from non-grass-fed sources
- An excess of hormones from foods, various health and beauty products, and plastic packaging
- Exposure to chemicals from household cleansers, computers, and microwaves
- Preservatives and food coloring
- Pesticides and herbicides
- Regular intake of processed and refined foods

You may be surprised by some of the foods that ended up on this list – certain proteins. But just because these may be classified as acidic, it does not mean that you should totally abstain from eating these foods.

 Your body still needs them in order to function effectively. Some of these foods consist of nutrients that are greatly beneficial like antioxidants and omega-3 fatty acids. These nutrients are vital for your body's development and overall health.

The alkaline diet is not about cutting a wide range of foods from your daily consumption and sticking to a minimal selection. No! Should you cut out foods that are important for your body's development, you will end up experiencing a number of health-related complications.

The alkaline diet is about achieving a balance that is healthy and beneficial for your body's general development. This stable and healthy kind of balance will allow your body to maintain a pH level that will benefit your health greatly. If your pH becomes too alkaline, which can happen, adding some acidic foods to your meals will be beneficial and healthy.

 Our problem is more about not taking in enough alkaline-promoting foods, instead of taking in too many acids from healthy, wholesome foods. You need to eat a wide variety of foods that are whole and organic, while avoiding regular consumption of foods that are processed and high in preservatives, saturated fats, and additives. This is the only ideal way to practically incorporate the alkaline diet into your life.

Chapter Two: One Week Meal Plan

This chapter is dedicated to assisting beginners with getting their alkaline diet started. If you struggle with meal planning, you can use this 7-day plan as a starting point. Some specialists recommend that beginners should start the diet with two alkaline meals (breakfast and lunch) and a late dinner. This meal plan involves three 3 alkaline meals a day – breakfast, lunch, and dinner. Some of the recipes may contain processed ingredients, dairy, etc. As I mentioned in the previous chapter, the Alkaline Diet is about balance. There is nothing wrong with consuming a few acidic ingredients every now and then. Some days will be repeated in order for the diet process to be as economic and convenient for you as possible

Day One

Breakfast: Non-Dairy Apple Parfait

A simple, nutrition-packed apple parfait to get your morning started the right way – and without the dairy.

Ingredients:

- ½ cup of soaked raw cashews (soak them for 20 mins- 1 hour prior to cooking)
- ½ cup of unsweetened almond or coconut milk
- ½ teaspoon of vanilla
- 1 cup of chopped apple pieces
- 1/3 cup of rolled oats – preferably gluten free and uncooked
- 1 tablespoon of hemp seeds

Directions:

Combine the cashews, almond or coconut milk, and the teaspoon of vanilla in a blender and blend until the mixture becomes smooth. Layer the ingredients in a small cup: heaping a spoon of cashew cream, spoonful of apples, top the layers with oats and hemp seeds and enjoy your breakfast.

Lunch: Savory Avocado Wrap

Ingredients required:

- 1 butter lettuce
- ½ of an avocado
- 1 teaspoon of basil, chopped
- Handful of spinach
- 1 teaspoon of chopped cilantro
- ¼ of red onion, diced
- 1 tomato, sliced
- Sea salt & ground, black pepper

Directions:

Spread avocado onto the lettuce. Sprinkle it with basil, cilantro, diced red onion, sliced tomato, sea salt and ground black pepper. Add the spinach, fold it in half and enjoy your meal!

Dinner: Thai Coconut Broccoli Soup

A flavorsome supper, like this Thai Coconut Broccoli Soup, is one of the best ways to end of your day.

Ingredients:

- 3 tablespoons of green curry paste
- 1 ½ cups of reduced fat coconut milk

- 2 cups of water
- 1 pound of broccoli, chopped
- 7 oz. of baby spinach, save some leaves for garnish
- Sea salt
- Freshly-ground pepper
- 1 spring onion, sliced
- Coriander leaves

<u>Directions</u>

Place the curry paste in a saucepan and allow it to cook, over medium heat, for one minute. Add the coconut milk and the water and bring the mixture to boil. Add broccoli and cook for ten minutes until it is tender. Add the spinach right after and allow to cook until your spinach has wilted (about 2 minutes). Switch off the heat, use a hand-held blender to blend the soup until it becomes smooth. Season to taste. This soup can serve 4 people. If you are less than four, you can freeze the remaining soup for a later time.

Breakfast: Crunch Berry Almond Butter Smoothie

It's sweet. It's tasty. It'll definitely be a repeat recipe on your list.

Ingredients:

- Spinach (2 cups, fresh)
- 2 cups of unsweetened almond milk
- Frozen berries (1 cup, mixed)
- 1 banana, frozen, chopped
- Almond butter (4 tbsp., raw)
- 1 tbsp. chia seeds

Directions:

First, place the almond milk and the spinach in the blender and blend. After this, add the almond butter, banana, and berries then blend until smooth. Add the chia seeds, reduce to a low speed, and continue blending to mix. Allow to rest for a few minutes, then enjoy.

Lunch: Kale and Cucumber Kimchi

You'll enjoy this nutrition-packed alkaline feast – and your body will be grateful for it too!

Ingredients:

- 1 Cup of thinly sliced white cabbage
- 1 Cup of chopped kale
- 1 Cup of diced cucumber
- 2 tablespoons of sea salt
- 1 tablespoon of paprika
- 1 tablespoon of finely chopped garlic

- 1 teaspoon of finely grated ginger
- 2 cups of filtered or alkaline water

Directions

Note: This dish should be prepared at least three days before you intend on eating it. Some people ferment their kimchi for months but if you are a beginner, this is not necessary.

Add the cabbage, kale, cucumber and salt together in a boil. Using your hands, squeeze the vegetables for 5 minutes. This will assist with releasing the vegetables' natural water. Stir the rest of the ingredients and move them to a jar – the jar must be sterilized. Cover the jar with its lid.

Leave the jar on your kitchen counter, away from any direct sunlight, for at least three days. As mentioned earlier, the mixture can be left to ferment for longer but this is not necessary. This can be eaten alone or on top of some cooked quinoa and roasted vegetables.

It's also normal for the mixture to have a bit of a smell – something close to sauerkraut.

Dinner: Pasta with Kale Pesto

A wholesome pasta meal to end of the day.

Ingredients:

- Kale (1 bunch)
- Basil (2 cups, fresh)
- Olive oil (1/4 cup, extra virgin)
- Walnuts (1/2 cup)
- Limes (2 small, juiced)
- Salt and pepper

- Zucchini (1, spiraled)
- Asparagus (sliced, for garnish)
- Spinach (leaves for garnish)
- Tomato (sliced for garnish)

Directions:

Set the walnuts to soak overnight so that its level of absorption improves.

When you are ready to prepare, add all your ingredients (except zucchini) into your blender, and pulse until creamy. Add your zucchini noodles to a bowl, pour the prepared sauce on top, stir and serve. Enjoy!

Breakfast: Oats with Apple and Almond Butter

This sweet, simple breakfast provides fiber, alkalinity and natural sugars. All the right ingredients to start your day.

Ingredients:

- 2 cups of oats – gluten-free
- 1 ½ cups almond or coconut milk
- 1/3 cup of raw almond butter
- 1 cup of grated green apple
- 1 teaspoon of cinnamon

Directions:

In a bowl, mix together the coconut or almond milk, oats, and almond butter. Stir in the grated apple. Cover the bowl with a plastic wrap. Place in the refrigerator and leave it overnight. If the oatmeal is too thick, just add more almond or coconut milk. Use cinnamon powder as garnish.

Lunch: The Green Bowl with Avocado Cumin Dressing

A healthy and tasty lunch to make your day!

Ingredients for the avocado cumin dressing:

- 1 avocado – medium to large sized
- 1 tablespoon of cumin powder
- 2 limes – freshly squeezed
- 1 cup of filtered or alkaline water
- ¼ teaspoon of sea salt
- 1 tablespoon of extra virgin olive oil
- A pinch of cayenne pepper
- You can also add ¼ teaspoon of smoked paprika

- <u>Ingredients for the Tahini Lemon Dressing:</u>
- ¼ cup of sesame butter (tahini)
- ½ cup filtered or alkaline water (more if you desire thinner dressing, less for thicker)
- ½ a medium-sized lemon, fresh squeezed
- 1 clove minced garlic
- ¾ teaspoon of sea salt (Celtic Gray, Himalayan, etc.)
- 1 tablespoon of extra virgin olive oil
- Freshly-ground black pepper to taste

<u>Ingredients for the salad:</u>

- 3 cups of chopped kale
- ½ cup of chopped broccoli florets
- ½ cup of zucchini (use a spiralizer to make noodles)
- ½ cup of noodles (kelp), soaked and drained
- 1/4 cup of halved cherry tomatoes
- 2 tbsp. of seeds (hemp)

<u>Directions:</u>

Steam broccoli and kale lightly for 4 mins. Set aside. Combine both the zucchini and noodles (kelp); toss them with a large serving of avocado dressing. Place cherry tomatoes in the mix and toss. In a plate, place the steamed kale and broccoli and drizzle over with the tahini dressing. Place tomatoes and dressed noodles atop kale and broccoli. Garnish with hemp seeds; enjoy your meal!

Dinner: Warm Avocado and Quinoa Salad

A nice warm salad to end a great day.

<u>Ingredients:</u>

- 4 ripe medium-sized avocados – peeled and cut into quarter pieces
- 1 cup of quinoa
- 1 14 oz. tin of chickpeas – drained
- 1 oz. of torn flat-leaf parsley

Directions:

Place two cups of water in a pot. Add the quinoa and bring to the boil. Allow to simmer on reduced heat. Place the lid on the pot and allow twelve minutes for cooking; or until water has evaporated. Quinoa can be tested by fluffing the grains with a fork. Grains should appear swollen and glassy.

Place all the ingredients in a bowl and toss thoroughly together. Use black pepper and sea salt to season the salad. Garnish salad with olive oil and lemon wedges.

Day Four

Breakfast: Crunch Berry Almond Butter Smoothie

It's sweet. It's tasty. It'll definitely be a repeat recipe on your list.

Ingredients:

- Spinach (2 cups, fresh)
- 2 cups of unsweetened almond milk
- Frozen berries (1 cup, mixed)
- 1 banana, frozen, chopped
- Almond butter (4 tbsp., raw)
- 1 tbsp. chia seeds

Directions:

First, place the almond milk and the spinach in the blender and blend. After this, add the almond butter, banana, and berries then blend until smooth. Add the chia seeds, reduce to a low speed, and continue blending to mix. Allow to rest for a few minutes, then enjoy.

Lunch: Kale and Cucumber Kimchi

You'll enjoy this nutrition-packed alkaline feast – and your body will be grateful for it too!

Ingredients:

- 1 Cup of thinly sliced white cabbage
- 1 Cup of chopped kale
- 1 Cup of diced cucumber
- 2 tablespoons of sea salt
- 1 tablespoon of paprika
- 1 tablespoon of finely chopped garlic

- 1 teaspoon of finely grated ginger
- 2 cups of filtered or alkaline water

Directions

Note: This dish should be prepared at least three days before you intend on eating it. Some people ferment their kimchi for months but if you are a beginner, this is not necessary.

Add the cabbage, kale, cucumber and salt together in a boil. Using your hands, squeeze the vegetables for 5 minutes. This will assist with releasing the vegetables' natural water. Stir the rest of the ingredients and move them to a jar – the jar must be sterilized. Cover the jar with its lid.

Leave the jar on your kitchen counter, away from any direct sunlight, for at least three days. As mentioned earlier, the mixture can be left to ferment for longer but this is not necessary. This can be eaten alone or on top of some cooked quinoa and roasted vegetables.

It's also normal for the mixture to have a bit of a smell – something close to sauerkraut.

Dinner: Pasta with Kale Pesto

A wholesome pasta meal to end of the day.

Ingredients:

- Kale (1 bunch)
- Basil (2 cups, fresh)
- Olive oil (1/4 cup, extra virgin)
- Walnuts (1/2 cup)
- Limes (2 small, juiced)
- Salt and pepper

- Zucchini (1, spiraled)
- Asparagus (sliced, for garnish)
- Spinach (leaves for garnish)
- Tomato (sliced for garnish)

Directions:

Set the walnuts to soak overnight so that its level of absorption improves.

When you are ready to prepare, add all your ingredients (except zucchini) into your blender, and pulse until creamy. Add your zucchini noodles to a bowl, pour the prepared sauce on top, stir and serve. Enjoy!

Breakfast: Non-Dairy Apple Parfait

A simple, nutrition-packed apple parfait to get your morning started the right way – and without the dairy.

Ingredients:

- ½ cup of soaked raw cashews (soak them for 20 mins- 1 hour prior to cooking)
- ½ cup of unsweetened almond or coconut milk
- ½ teaspoon of vanilla
- 1 cup of chopped apple pieces
- 1/3 cup of rolled oats – preferably gluten free and uncooked
- 1 tablespoon of hemp seeds

Directions:

Combine the cashews, almond or coconut milk, and the teaspoon of vanilla in a blender and blend until the mixture becomes smooth. Layer the ingredients in a small cup: heaping a spoon of cashew cream, spoonful of apples, top the layers with oats and hemp seeds and enjoy your breakfast.

Lunch: Savory Avocado Wrap

Ingredients required:

- 1 butter lettuce
- ½ of an avocado
- 1 teaspoon of basil, chopped
- Handful of spinach
- 1 teaspoon of chopped cilantro

- ¼ of red onion, diced
- 1 tomato, sliced
- Sea salt & ground, black pepper

Directions:

Spread avocado onto the lettuce. Sprinkle it with basil, cilantro, diced red onion, sliced tomato, sea salt and ground black pepper. Add the spinach, fold it in half and enjoy your meal!

Dinner: Thai Coconut Broccoli Soup

A flavorsome supper, like this Thai Coconut Broccoli Soup, is one of the best ways to end of your day.

Ingredients:

- 3 tablespoons of green curry paste
- 1 ½ cups of reduced fat coconut milk
- 2 cups of water
- 1 pound of broccoli, chopped
- 7 oz. of baby spinach, save some leaves for garnish
- Sea salt
- Freshly-ground pepper
- 1 spring onion, sliced
- Coriander leaves

Directions

Place the curry paste in a saucepan and allow it to cook, over medium heat, for one minute. Add the coconut milk and the water and bring the mixture to boil. Add broccoli and cook for ten minutes until it is tender. Add the spinach right after and cook for a couple of minutes, or until the spinach wilts.

Remove the pan from the heat and use a hand-held blender to blend the soup until it becomes smooth. Season it with salt and pepper. This soup can serve 4 people. If you are less than four, you can freeze the remaining soup for a later time.

Breakfast: Oats with Apple and Almond Butter

This sweet, simple breakfast provides fiber, alkalinity and natural sugars. All the right ingredients to start your day.

Ingredients:

- 2 cups of oats – gluten-free
- 1 ½ cups almond or coconut milk
- 1/3 cup of raw almond butter
- 1 cup of grated green apple
- 1 teaspoon of cinnamon

Directions:

In a bowl, mix together the coconut or almond milk, oats, and almond butter. Stir in the grated apple. Cover the bowl with a plastic wrap. Place in the refrigerator and leave it overnight. If the oatmeal is too thick, just add more almond or coconut milk. Use cinnamon powder as garnish.

Lunch: The Green Bowl with Avocado Cumin Dressing

A healthy and tasty lunch to make your day!

Ingredients for the avocado cumin dressing:

- 1 avocado – medium to large sized
- 1 tablespoon of cumin powder
- 2 limes – freshly squeezed
- 1 cup of filtered or alkaline water
- ¼ teaspoon of sea salt
- 1 tablespoon of extra virgin olive oil
- A pinch of cayenne pepper
- You can also add ¼ teaspoon of smoked paprika

- <u>Ingredients for the Tahini Lemon Dressing:</u>
- ¼ cup of sesame butter (tahini)
- ½ cup filtered or alkaline water (more if you desire thinner dressing, less for thicker)
- ½ a medium-sized lemon, fresh squeezed
- 1 clove minced garlic
- ¾ teaspoon of sea salt (Celtic Gray, Himalayan, etc.)
- 1 tablespoon of extra virgin olive oil
- Freshly-ground black pepper to taste

<u>Ingredients for the salad:</u>

- 3 cups of chopped kale
- ½ cup of chopped broccoli florets
- ½ cup of zucchini (use a spiralizer to make noodles)
- ½ cup of noodles (kelp), soaked and drained
- 1/4 cup of halved cherry tomatoes
- 2 tbsp. of seeds (hemp)

<u>Directions:</u>

Steam broccoli and kale lightly for 4 mins. Set aside. Combine both the zucchini and noodles (kelp); toss them with a large serving of avocado dressing. Place cherry tomatoes in the mix and toss. In a plate, place the steamed kale and broccoli and drizzle over with the tahini dressing. Place tomatoes and dressed noodles atop kale and broccoli. Garnish with hemp seeds; enjoy your meal!

Dinner: Warm Avocado and Quinoa Salad

A nice warm salad to end a great day.

<u>Ingredients:</u>

- 4 ripe medium-sized avocados – peeled and cut into quarter pieces
- 1 cup of quinoa
- 1 14 oz. tin of chickpeas – drained
- 1 oz. of torn flat-leaf parsley

<u>Directions:</u>

Place two cups of water in a pot. Add the quinoa and bring to the boil. Allow to simmer on reduced heat. Place the lid on the pot and allow twelve minutes for cooking; or until water has evaporated. Quinoa can be tested by fluffing the grains with a fork. Grains should appear swollen and glassy.

Place all the ingredients in a bowl and toss thoroughly together. Use black pepper and sea salt to season the salad. Garnish salad with olive oil and lemon wedges.

Breakfast: Crunch Berry Almond Butter Smoothie

It's sweet. It's tasty. It'll definitely be a repeat recipe on your list.

Ingredients:

- Spinach (2 cups, fresh)
- 2 cups of unsweetened almond milk
- Frozen berries (1 cup, mixed)
- 1 banana, frozen, chopped
- Almond butter (4 tbsp., raw)
- 1 tbsp. chia seeds

Directions:

First, place the almond milk and the spinach in the blender and blend. After this, add the almond butter, banana, and berries then blend until smooth. Add the chia seeds, reduce to a low speed, and continue blending to mix. Allow to rest for a few minutes, then enjoy.

Lunch: Kale and Cucumber Kimchi

You'll enjoy this nutrition-packed alkaline feast – and your body will be grateful for it too!

Ingredients:

- 1 Cup of thinly sliced white cabbage
- 1 Cup of chopped kale
- 1 Cup of diced cucumber
- 2 tablespoons of sea salt
- 1 tablespoon of paprika
- 1 tablespoon of finely chopped garlic

- 1 teaspoon of finely grated ginger
- 2 cups of filtered or alkaline water

<u>Directions</u>

Note: This dish should be prepared at least three days before you intend on eating it. Some people ferment their kimchi for months but if you are a beginner, this is not necessary.

Add the cabbage, kale, cucumber and salt together in a boil. Using your hands, squeeze the vegetables for 5 minutes. This will assist with releasing the vegetables' natural water. Stir the rest of the ingredients and move them to a jar – the jar must be sterilized. Cover the jar with its lid.

Leave the jar on your kitchen counter, away from any direct sunlight, for at least three days. As mentioned earlier, the mixture can be left to ferment for longer but this is not necessary. This can be eaten alone or on top of some cooked quinoa and roasted vegetables.

It's also normal for the mixture to have a bit of a smell – something close to sauerkraut.

Dinner: Pasta with Kale Pesto

A wholesome pasta meal to end of the day.

<u>Ingredients:</u>

- Kale (1 bunch)
- Basil (2 cups, fresh)
- Olive oil (1/4 cup, extra virgin)
- Walnuts (1/2 cup)
- Limes (2 small, juiced)
- Salt and pepper

- Zucchini (1, spiraled)
- Asparagus (sliced, for garnish)
- Spinach (leaves for garnish)
- Tomato (sliced for garnish)

Directions:

Set the walnuts to soak overnight so that its level of absorption improves.

When you are ready to prepare, add all your ingredients (except zucchini) into your blender, and pulse until creamy. Add your zucchini noodles to a bowl, pour the prepared sauce on top, stir and serve. Enjoy!

Chapter Three: Breakfast Alkaline Diet Recipes

Berry Almond Butter Smoothie

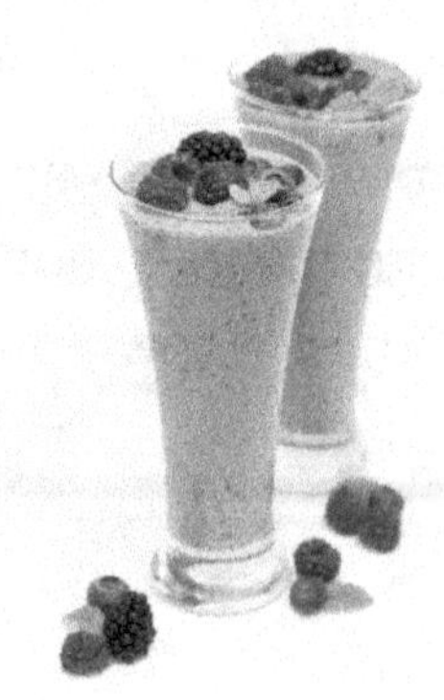

Ingredients:

- 1 cup spinach
- 0.5 cups mixed berries
- 2 tablespoons almond butter
- 1 cup almond milk
- 1 frozen banana

Directions:

1. Blend the almond milk and spinach.
2. Once liquefied, add the other ingredients.
3. Blend until it's smooth.
4. If you want to add a bit of crunch, toss in a serving of chia seeds.

Nutritional Information per Serving:

Calories: 174; Total Fat: 2.4g; Carbs: 38g; Protein: 1.8g

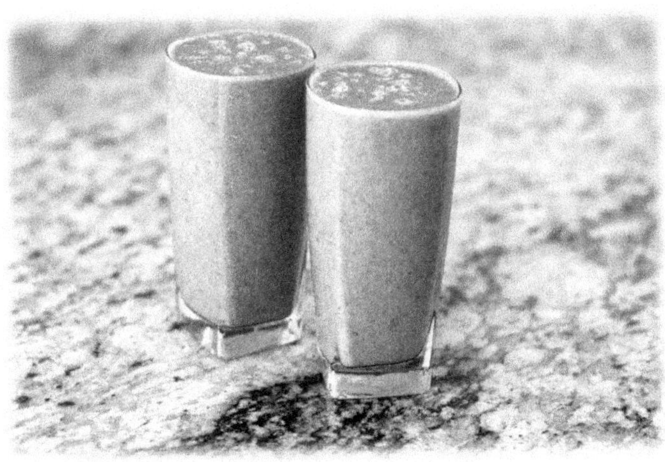

Ingredients:

- 1 cucumber
- 1-inch ginger, fresh
- 1 pear
- 0.5 lemon
- 0.5 handful string beans
- 1 tablespoon chia seeds

Directions:

1. Juice the lemon and cucumber.
2. Juice the pear and string beans.
3. Mix well and juice the ginger.
4. Before serving, sprinkle chia seeds.

Nutritional Information per Serving:

Calories: 182.3; Total Fat: 1.5g; Carbs: 42.9g; Protein: 6g

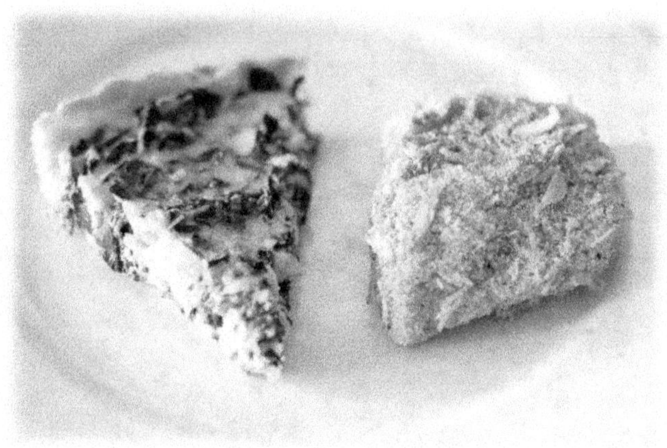

Ingredients:

- 2 tablespoons olive oil
- 2 leeks
- 1 bunch kale
- 0.5 teaspoons coriander
- 6 eggs
- 0.5 teaspoons cumin
- 60 grams feta
- 0.025 cups pine nuts
- 1 shallot
- 1 bunch Swiss chard
- 0.5 lemon zest
- 1 pinch chili flakes
- 100 grams mozzarella
- Pepper and salt

Directions:

1. Chop the shallots, dice the leeks, zest the lemon half and grate the mozzarella.
2. Preheat the oven to 180 °F.

3. Remove the stems from the vegetables.
4. Layer all leaves and create tight rolls before slicing into strips.
5. In a pan, cook the shallots.
6. Cook the leeks.
7. Add the kale and chard.
8. Cook until they soften.
9. Add the spices and zest.
10. Separately mix the eggs, cooked vegetables, and both kinds of cheese.
11. Pour into the pan for the oven.
12. Sprinkle pine nuts.
13. Bake for 15 minutes, covered.
14. Bake for an additional 20 minutes, uncovered.
15. Serve and enjoy.

Nutritional Information per Serving:

Calories: 191; Total Fat: 13.6g; Carbs: 6g; Protein: 12g

Quinoa Porridge

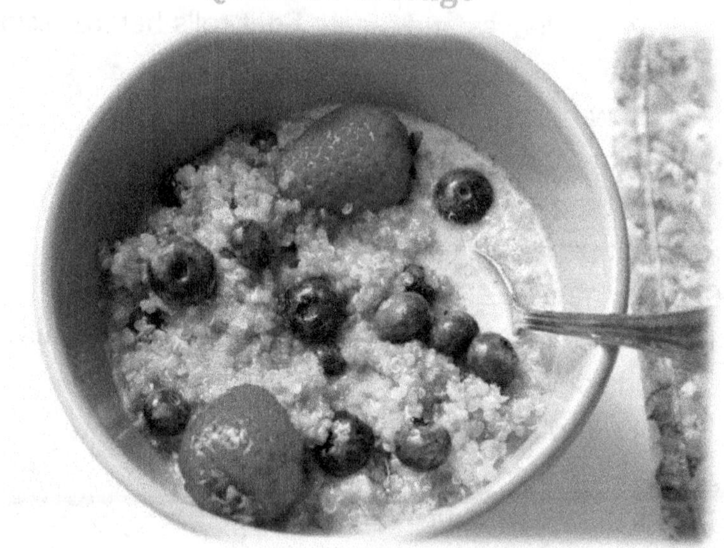

Ingredients:

- 0.5 cups quinoa
- 1 teaspoon cinnamon
- 1 teaspoon hemp seeds
- 15 ounces coconut milk
- 1 teaspoon chia seeds

Directions:

1. In a pan, place all ingredients, except hemp seeds.
2. Cook for 10 to 15 minutes.
3. Sprinkle hemp seeds all over.

Nutritional Information per Serving:

Calories: 265.5; Total Fat: 5.8g; Carbs: 45.7g; Protein: 8.4g

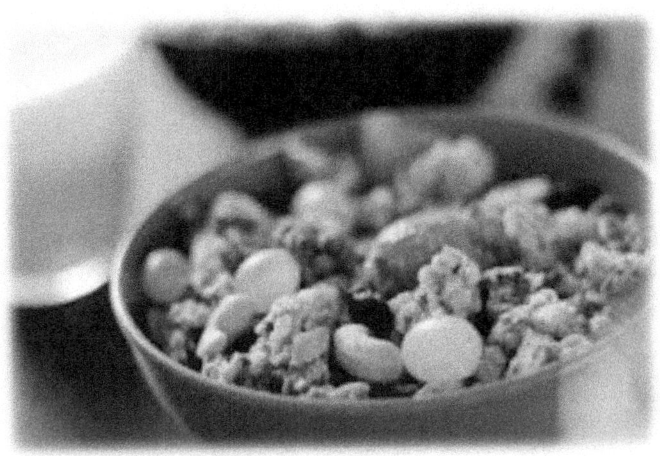

Ingredients:

- 0.5 cups oats that contain no gluten
- 1 tablespoon almonds, sliced
- Dash of cinnamon
- 1 cup coconut milk that is not sweetened
- 0.5 cups apple

Directions:

1. Dice the apple.
2. Portion and combine ingredients.
3. Soak the ingredients and put them in the refrigerator, store overnight.
4. Simply heat for approximately two minutes in the morning

Nutritional Information per Serving:

Calories: 161; Total Fat: 3.2g; Carbs: 25.5g; Protein: 4.8g

Banana Coco Shake

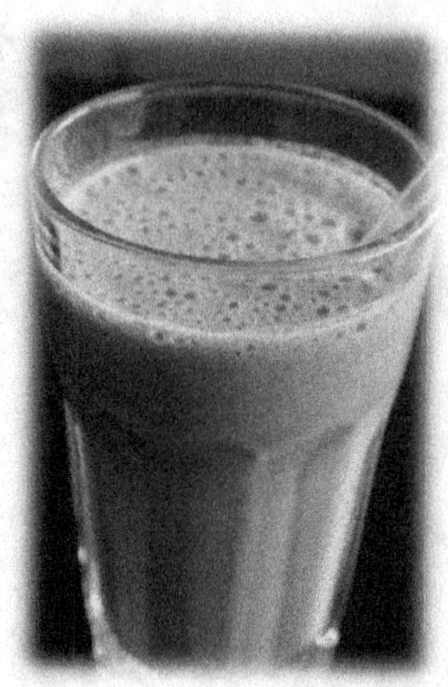

Ingredients:

- 1 frozen banana
- 0.5 scoop almond butter
- 0.5 teaspoons coconut nectar
- 0.5 cups coconut milk
- 0.5 tablespoons coconut oil
- Dash cinnamon
- 2 tablespoons chia seeds

Directions:

1. Place all ingredients, except seeds and cinnamon, into a blender.
2. Blend until you get the consistency that you prefer.
3. Add in chia seeds and mix for a few more seconds to disperse them.
4. Sprinkle cinnamon on top.

Nutritional Information per Serving:

Calories: 208; Total Fat: 1.52g; Carbs: 47.9g; Protein: 4.77g

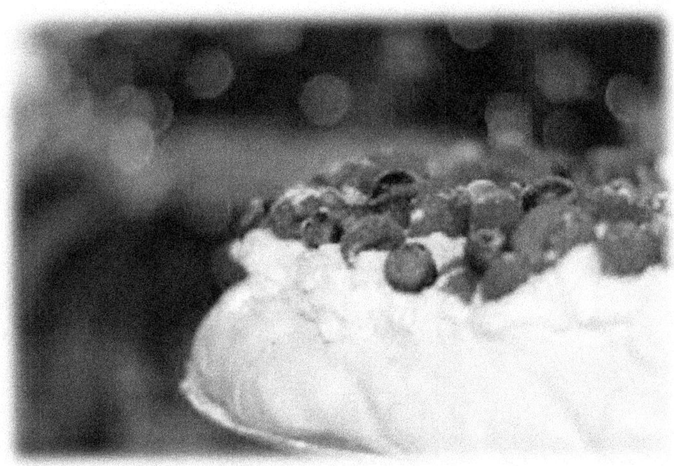

Ingredients:

- 1 cup mixed berries
- 1 tablespoon mint
- 2 tablespoons coconut butter

Directions:

1. Chop the mint.
2. Melt the coconut butter.
3. Place berries in a bowl.
4. Add the mint and mix.
5. Pour melted butter over berries.

Nutritional Information per Serving:

Calories: 53; Total Fat: 4.7g; Carbs: 2.3g; Protein: 0.6g

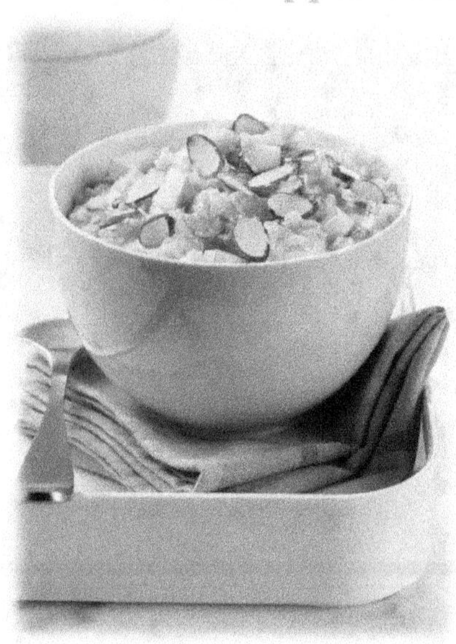

Ingredients:

- 1 cups oats that do not contain gluten
- 0.33 almond butter
- 1 teaspoon cinnamon
- 1.5 cups coconut milk
- 1 cup green apple

Directions:

1. Grate the apple.
2. Put the butter, milk, and oats in a bowl after mixing it up with the apple.
3. Cover and refrigerate.
4. In the morning, heat the oats.
5. Top with cinnamon.

Nutritional Information per Serving:

Calories: 330; Total Fat: 12g; Carbs: 53g; Protein: 9g

Strawberry Quinoa

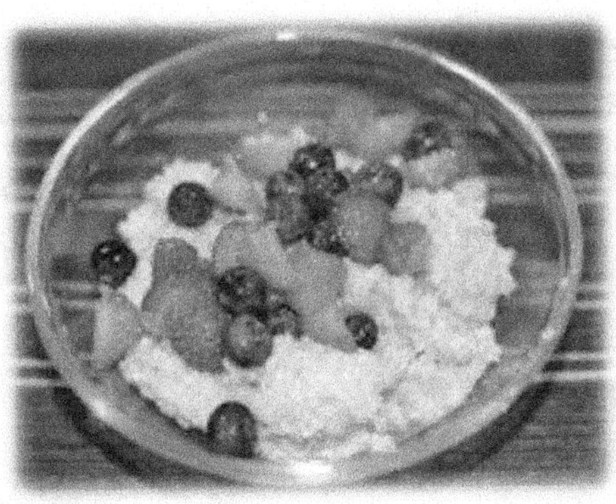

Ingredients:

- 1 cup quinoa
- 1.5 cups almond milk
- 2 pitted dates
- 2 tablespoons coconut flakes that do not have added sweetener
- 5 tablespoons chia seeds
- 0.5 cups strawberries
- 2 tablespoons almonds

Directions:

1. Cook the quinoa as per instructions.
2. Quarter the strawberries.
3. Chop the almonds.
4. Combine the strawberries, dates and almond milk, and purée.
5. Put chia seeds in a jar and mix with the purée.
6. Place in a bowl and add shredded coconut and quinoa.
7. Place an additional quartered strawberry as garnish.

Nutritional Information per Serving:

Calories: 217; Total Fat: 9g; Carbs: 28g; Protein: 7g

Apple Parfait

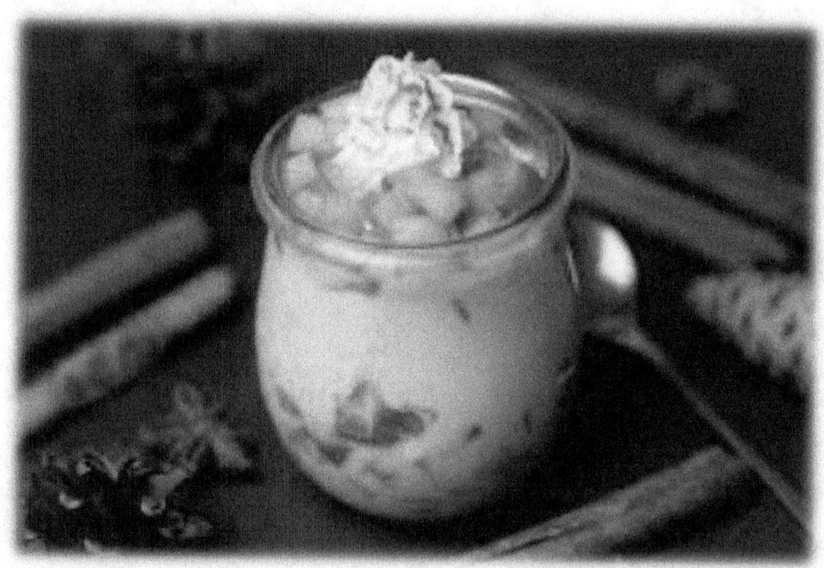

Ingredients:

- 0.5 cups raw cashews
- 0.5 teaspoons vanilla
- 0.33 cups oats that are free from gluten
- 0.5 cups almond milk that is not sweetened
- 1 cup apple
- 1 tablespoon hemp seeds

Directions:

1. Blend almond milk, cashews, and vanilla.
2. In a cup, place the puree and apples.
3. Top with hemp seeds and oats.

Nutritional Information per Serving:

Calories: 295; Total Fat: 7g; Carbs: 55.4g; Protein: 6.6g

Chapter Four: Main Dishes Alkaline Diet Recipes

Summer Minestrone Soup

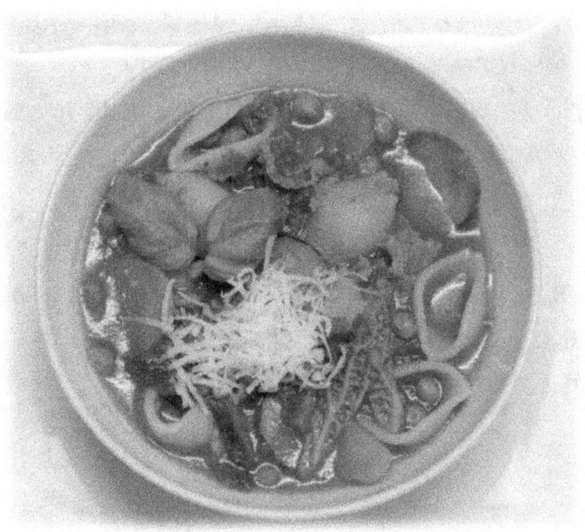

Ingredients:

- Pepper
- Himalayan salt
- 2 cloves minced garlic
- 1 cup /240 ml fresh corn kernels
- ½ cup /120 ml frozen peas
- 4 cups /.95 L low-sodium vegetable broth
- 1 large chopped onion
- 1 small chopped carrot
- ½ bunch basil
- 1 tbsp. /15 ml olive oil
- 1 small chopped yellow squash
- 1 small chopped zucchini
- 8 oz. /224 g red potatoes

Directions:

1. Heat oil in a pan. Add onion and sprinkle with pepper and salt.
2. Cover and simmer until onions turn translucent.
3. Uncover and allow to cook until the onions have become tender and browned slightly.
4. Chop 1 tablespoon basil stems and add to onions and garlic. Add broth and potatoes. Simmer 5 minutes.
5. Add carrot, squash, and zucchini. Simmer 3 minutes. Add corn and peas. Continue to cook until veggies are tender.
6. Serve the soup with a sprinkle of basil.

Nutritional Information per Serving:

Calories: 153; Total Fat: 3.1g; Carbs: 29.1g; Protein: 6.2g

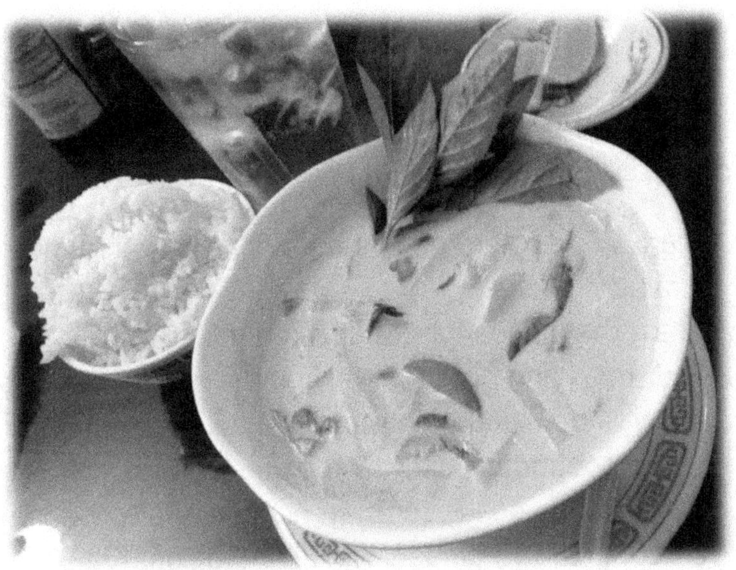

Ingredients:

<u>Curry:</u>

- Pepper
- Salt
- 1 cup /240 ml veggie stock
- 2 14-oz /396 g cans coconut milk
- Pinch cayenne (optional)
- 1 tbsp. /8 g curry powder
- 1/3 cup /28 g snow peas
- 1 tbsp. /15 ml coconut oil
- ¼ cup /45 g diced tomatoes
- ½ cup /64 g diced carrots
- ½ cup /45 g broccoli florets
- 1 tbsp. /6 g grated ginger
- 4 cloves minced garlic
- 1 small onion, diced

<u>Quinoa:</u>

- 1 cup /170 g quinoa, rinsed
- 1 14-oz /396 g can coconut milk
- 1 tbsp. /15 ml agave

Directions:

1. Start by prepping the quinoa by rinsing it in a mesh strainer.
2. Toast the quinoa for about three minutes.
3. Pour in a can of coconut milk and a half cup of water. Allow to boil, and then reduce to a simmer.
4. Cover pot and let cook 15 minutes.
5. While the quinoa is cooking, heat oil and sauté the broccoli, carrot, ginger, garlic, and onion.
6. Season to your liking with pepper and salt. Stir frequently until the veggies have softened, around five minutes.
7. Mix in another pinch of salt, coconut milk, veggie stock, cayenne, and curry powder. Let the mixture simmer for about ten to 15 minutes.
8. Stir in the tomatoes and snow peas during the last five minutes. Adjust the taste as needed, adding more pepper or salt.
9. Serve the curry over a helping of the coconut quinoa. Garnish with any herbs that you would like, and squeeze on some fresh lemon juice.

Nutritional Information per Serving:

Calories: 950; Total Fat: 63g; Carbs: 4.7g; Protein: 57.4g

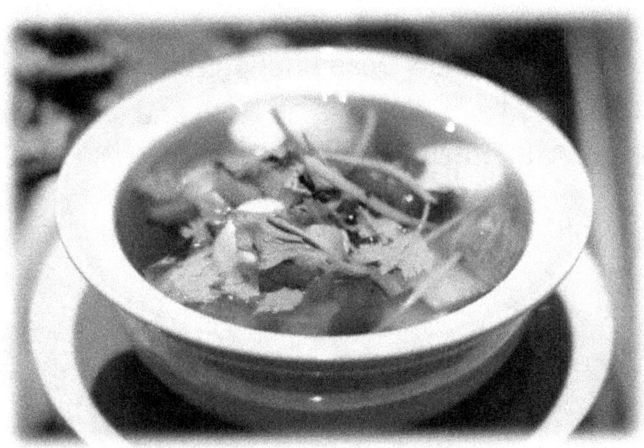

Ingredients:

- Himalayan salt
- 1 tsp /5 ml Thai red curry paste
- 1 tsp /5 ml grated fresh ginger
- 2 cups /470 ml low-sodium vegetable broth
- 4 oz. /112 g snow peas
- ¼ cup /60 ml torn basil leaves
- 1 14 oz. can /392 g coconut milk
- 14 oz. /392 g extra-firm tofu, drained and cubed
- 2 tbsp. /30 ml fresh lime juice
- ½ lb. /227 g mushrooms, sliced thin
- 2 carrots, halved lengthwise, sliced into half moons
- 4 oz. /112 g green beans, halved
- Asian chili garlic sauce

Directions:

1. Mix the curry paste and ginger together in a pot. Pour in the broth and coconut milk along with a teaspoon of salt. Whisk until smooth and bring to a boil.

2. Add mushrooms, carrots, and green beans. Simmer until tender.
3. Add tofu and snow peas until peas turn bright green.
4. Stir in lime juice. Sprinkle on basil and chili garlic sauce.

Nutritional Information per Serving:

Calories: 114.4; Total Fat: 3.6g; Carbs: 19.5g; Protein: 3.3g

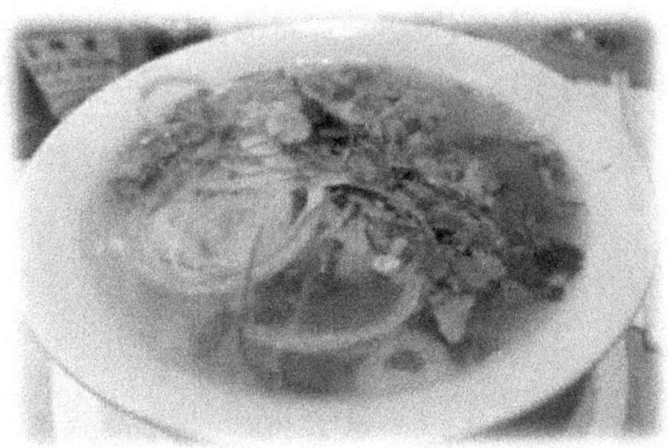

Ingredients:

- 8-oz /224 g bean sprouts
- 14-oz /392 g rice noodles, cooked
- 2 tsp /10 ml sesame oil
- 2 jalapeno peppers, sliced
- 6 oz. /168 g shiitake mushrooms stems removed
- 6 green onions, sliced
- 1 ½ tbsp. /22.5 ml vegan butter
- Salt
- 1 ½ tbsp. /22.5 ml hoisin sauce
- 1 tbsp. /15 ml grated ginger
- 64 oz. /1796 g vegetable broth

Directions:

1. Mix the salt, ginger, onion, and broth in a large pot. Allow to come to a rolling boil. Turn down the heat and allow to simmer for 15 minutes.
2. As the broth cooks, warm the butter in a skillet. Sauté the mushrooms for around six minutes. Mix in the sesame oil and hoisin sauce. Cook until everything has thickened and the mushrooms are coated. Take it off the heat.

3. Place the cooked noodles in four to six bowls. Fill each
    of the bowls with some of the broth. Top with cilantro,
    basil, mushrooms, jalapenos, and bean sprouts. Serve
    the pho with chili garlic sauce, hoisin, and a lime
    wedge.

Nutritional Information per Serving:

Calories: 290; Total Fat: 5.5g; Carbs: 42g; Protein: 16g

Coconut and Corn Soup

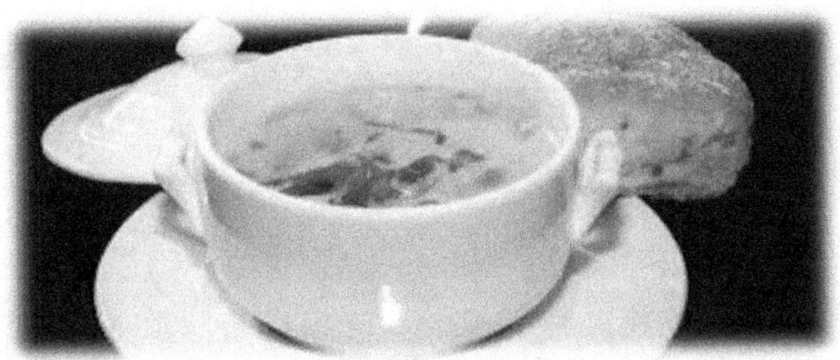

Ingredients:

- Pepper
- Himalayan salt
- 1 tbsp. /15 ml fresh lime juice
- 2 ½ cups /600 ml water
- 3 cups /720 ml fresh corn kernels
- 1 jalapeno chili, seeded and chopped
- 1 14 oz. can /392 g light coconut milk

Directions

1. Add water, coconut milk, corn kernels, and jalapeno to pot. Bring to boil. Simmer until corn is tender.
2. Use immersion blender to puree soup. Strain through sieve and discard solids. Season mixture to your taste.
3. Allow it to chill for three hours or overnight. Add lime juice. Stir. Garnish with fresh corn and sprinkle each serving with pepper.

Nutritional Information per Serving:

Calories: 170; Total Fat: 13g; Carbs: 13g; Protein: 2g

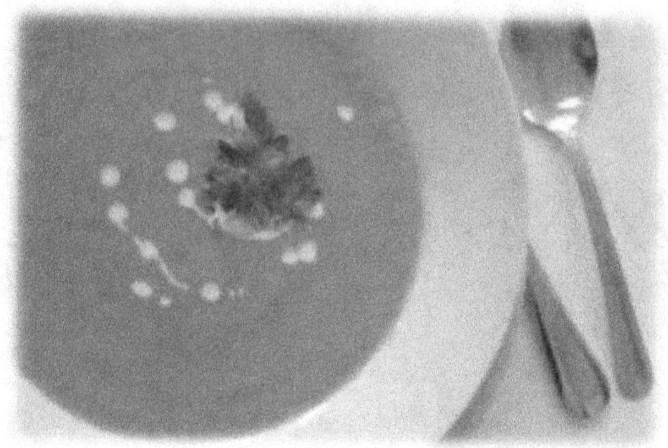

Ingredients:

- ½ tsp /2 ½ ml coriander
- Pepper
- ½ tsp /2 ½ ml cinnamon
- Salt
- 6 tbsp. /180 ml olive oil
- ¼ tsp /1 ¼ ml cayenne pepper
- 5 cups /1.2 L vegetable broth
- 1 tsp /5 ml cumin
- 3 cups /720 ml cooked carrots
- ½ cup /120 ml toasted pumpkin seeds
- ¼ tsp /1 ¼ ml allspice

Directions:

1. Add the carrots and broth to blender. Puree until smooth.
2. Put mixture in a pot. Add in salt and spices. Cook about 8 minutes. Add water until it is at the desired consistency.

3. Serve soup with pumpkin seeds, ground pepper, and
    drizzle with olive oil.

Nutritional Information per Serving:

Calories: 175.5; Total Fat: 8.2g; Carbs: 22.6g; Protein: 5.8g

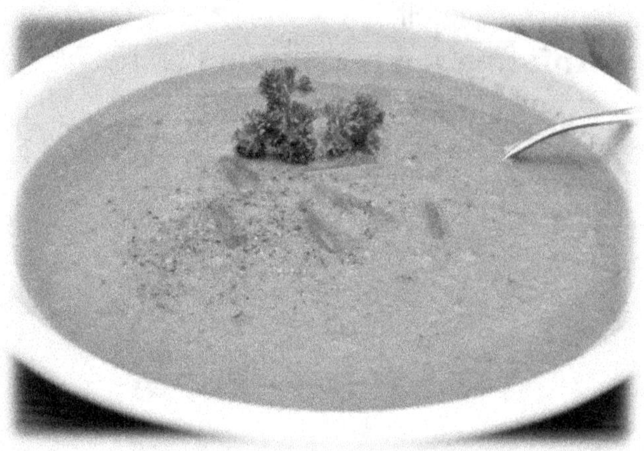

Ingredients:

- Pepper
- Himalayan salt
- Roasted peanuts, chopped
- Cilantro
- ½ cup /120 ml creamy peanut butter
- 2 tbsp. /30 ml olive oil
- 4 garlic cloves, minced
- 1 15 oz. /420 g diced tomatoes
- 2 tsp /10 ml cumin
- 1 large chopped onion
- 1 ½ lb. /680 g sweet potatoes, peeled and chopped
- ¼ tsp /1 ¼ ml cayenne
- 2 tbsp. /30 ml fresh grated ginger

Directions

1. Heat oil in a pan. Add onion, season with pepper and salt. Cover and cook until tender.
2. Add ginger and garlic. Stir. Add cayenne and cumin. Stir. Add sweet potatoes and stir to combine.

3. Add water, peanut butter, and tomatoes. Allow the water to boil. Cover and allow to cook until sweet potatoes can easily be pierced with a fork.
4. Serve the soup with peanuts and cilantro.

Nutritional Information per Serving:

Calories: 269.3; Total Fat: 9.1g; Carbs: 35.5g; Protein: 11g

Breakfast Miso Soup

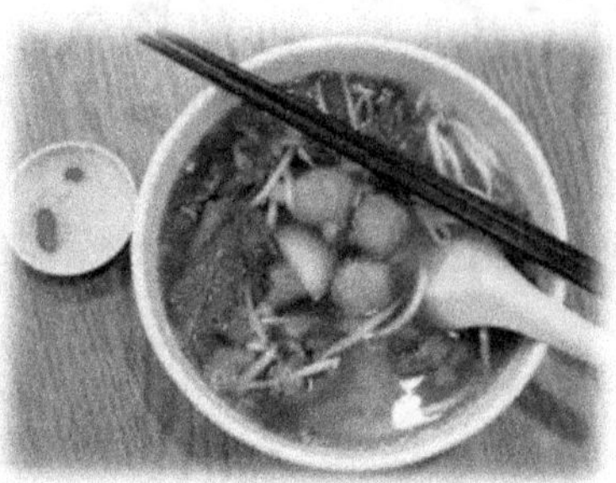

Ingredients:

- Pepper
- Salt
- 2 tbsp. /30 ml olive oil
- ½ chopped onion
- 2 minced garlic cloves
- 2 tbsp. /30 ml white miso
- 1 cup /240 ml broccoli florets
- 2 diced celery stalks
- 1 cup /240 ml cooked chickpeas
- 2 peeled and diced carrots

Directions

1. Heat oil in pan. Add onion, carrots, celery, and garlic. Let sauté until the veggies become tender.
2. Mix in chickpeas and broccoli. Cook for two minutes.
3. Add four cups water. Allow to come to a boil. Cook until veggies are tender. Take off heat. Add in the miso and stir until dissolved. Taste and add pepper and salt as needed.

Nutritional Information per Serving:

Calories: 84; Total Fat: 3.36g; Carbs: 7.78g; Protein: 6.02g

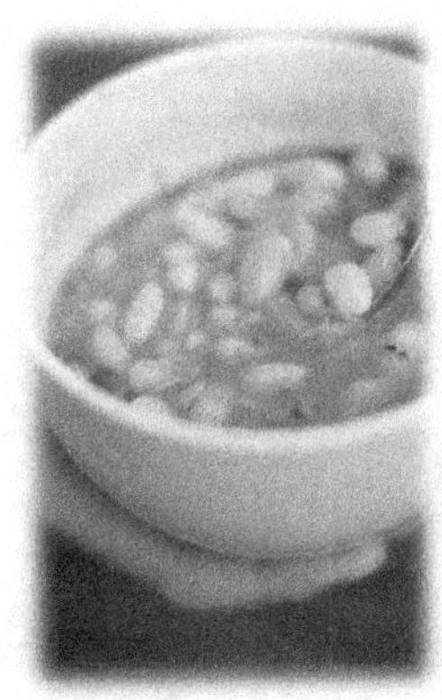

Ingredients:

- 1 ½ tsp /7 ml lemon juice
- Pepper
- Himalayan salt
- 1 clove minced garlic
- 2 tsp /10 ml olive oil
- 2 thinly sliced scallions
- 1 15 oz. /420 g can white beans, rinsed and drained
- ½ tsp / 2 ½ ml oregano

Directions:

1. Heat oil in pan. Add oregano, garlic, and scallions. Sauté until soft.
2. Add beans and broth. Stir. Cook until hot.
3. Mash beans with spoon or potato masher to help thicken soup.
4. Add lemon juice. Stir well. Season with pepper and salt. Enjoy.

Nutritional Information per Serving:

Calories: 150; Total Fat: 0.5g; Carbs: 28g; Protein: 7g

Loaded Veggie Soup

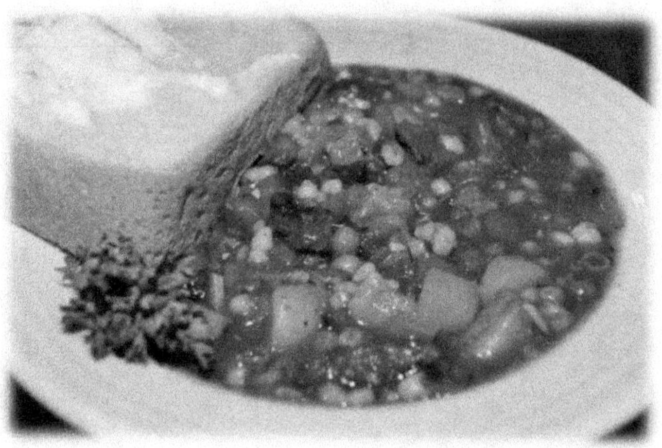

Ingredients:

- Pepper
- Himalayan salt
- 3 15 oz./420 g cannellini beans
- 1 cup /240 ml frozen peas
- 1 15 oz. /420 g diced tomatoes
- 8 oz. /224 g broccoli rabe, remove thick stems
- 1 large chopped onion
- 1 medium chopped zucchini
- 6 garlic cloves, minced
- ½ small butternut squash
- 2 tsp /10 ml Italian seasoning
- 1 fennel bulb or 4 celery stalks

Directions:

1. Work in batches if you need to. Puree beans and tomatoes with juices. Pour into pot.
2. Add 4 cups water, pepper and salt to taste, Italian seasoning, garlic, and onion. Bring to a boil and allow it to cook for ten minutes.

3. Place in broccoli rabe, zucchini, squash, and fennel. Simmer vegetables until soft, around 20 minutes. Mix in peas and let them heat through.
4. Serve drizzled with oil.

Nutritional Information per Serving:

Calories: 150; Total Fat: 0.5g; Carbs: 28g; Protein: 7g

Chickpea Vegetable Soup

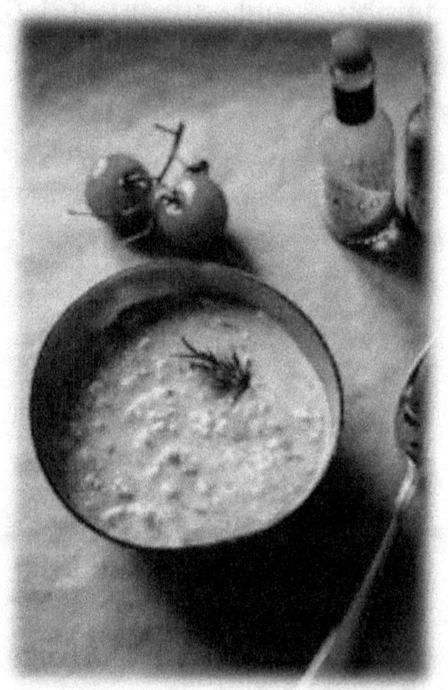

Ingredients:

- Pepper
- Salt
- 1 tbsp. /15 ml vegan margarine
- 3 cups /720 ml low-sodium vegetable broth
- 1 medium chopped onion
- ½ tsp /2 ½ ml turmeric
- 4 minced garlic cloves
- 1 cup /240 ml water
- 3 carrots, sliced into rounds
- 1 14.5 oz. /406 g diced tomatoes
- 4 celery stalks, sliced thin
- 2 tbsp. /30 ml olive oil
- 2 15 oz. /420 g cans chickpeas, drained and rinsed
- 1 bay leaf

Directions:

1. Heat oil and margarine in a pot.
2. Add bay leaf, garlic, celery, carrots, onions, pepper, and salt. Cook until veggies are tender.
3. Add tomatoes, chickpeas, and turmeric.
4. Add water and broth. Stir to combine. Bring to boil.
5. Allow it to simmer for ten minutes. Take off heat.
6. Taste and adjust seasonings if needed.
7. Serve, garnished with parsley.

Nutritional Information per Serving:

Calories: 90.7; Total Fat: 0.7g; Carbs: 17.9g; Protein: 3.8g

Rice Noodle Soup

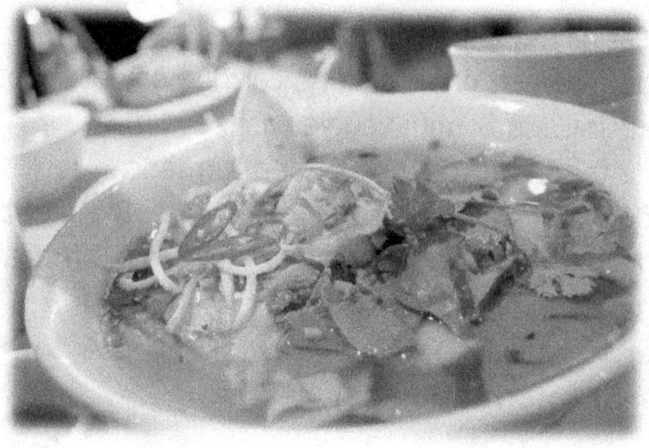

Ingredients:

- Lime wedge
- 2 tsp /10 ml salt
- Jalapeno, sliced
- Seasonal vegetables
- 1 tbsp. /30 ml vegetable oil
- Fried tofu cubes, optional
- ¼ c /60 ml red bell pepper, sliced
- 2 garlic cloves, chopped
- ¼ c /60 ml cremini mushrooms, sliced
- ¼ tsp /1.25 ml pepper
- 1 small onion, chopped
- 7 oz. /196 g dried vermicelli rice noodles

Directions:

1. Begin by prepping the noodles. Put the noodles in six cups of boiling water. Allow to sit, covered, for two minutes.
2. Drain them and rinse in cold water.

3. Begin frying the onion in a pan until they have become golden, about two minutes. Stir in garlic and allow the mixture to cook for 30 minutes.

4. Pour in six cups of boiling water, add pepper and salt.

5. As the broth simmers, chop up the herbs, pepper, and mushrooms.

6. Mix in the herbs, pepper, mushrooms, and any other seasonal vegetables that you want to the broth.

7. Allow this to simmer for a couple of minutes, or until you like the tenderness of the vegetables.

8. Take off of the heat.

9. Place some rice noodles in a bowl and ladle on some of the broth. Top with lime wedge and jalapeno.

Nutritional Information per Serving:

Calories: 222.1; Total Fat: 0g; Carbs: 51g; Protein: 4g

Creamy Vegetable Soup

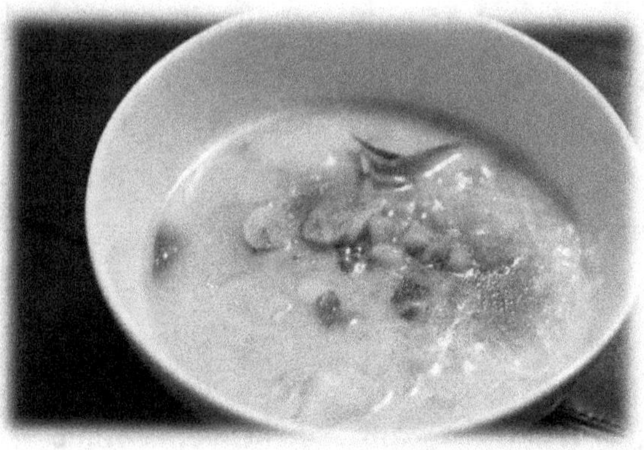

Ingredients:

- Pepper
- Salt
- 1 tbsp. /15 ml olive oil
- ¼ cup /60 ml coconut milk
- 3 sprigs fresh thyme
- 3 medium red potatoes, chunked
- 4 celery stalks, cut into ½-inch pieces
- 3 garlic cloves, halved
- 3 cups /720 ml vegetable stock
- 1 lb.454 g carrots, peeled cut into ½-inch pieces
- ¼ tsp /1 ¼ ml red pepper flakes
- 1 large chopped onion
- 2 bay leaves

Directions:

1. Heat oil in pan. Add celery, carrots, and onions. Add ½ tsp. salt and red pepper flakes. Cook until soft.
2. Add potatoes, thyme, bay leaves, and garlic. Cook about 5 minutes. You may add oil if the pan gets too dry.

3. Add stock and boil. Simmer until potatoes are fork tender.
4. Take soup off heat. Remove thyme sprigs and bay leaves and discard. Use an immersion blender and mix until you get a smooth consistency.
5. Mix in the coconut milk. Adjust seasoning if needed.

Nutritional Information per Serving:

Calories: 216; Total Fat: 7.8g; Carbs: 28.8g; Protein: 5.4g

Vegetable Momos

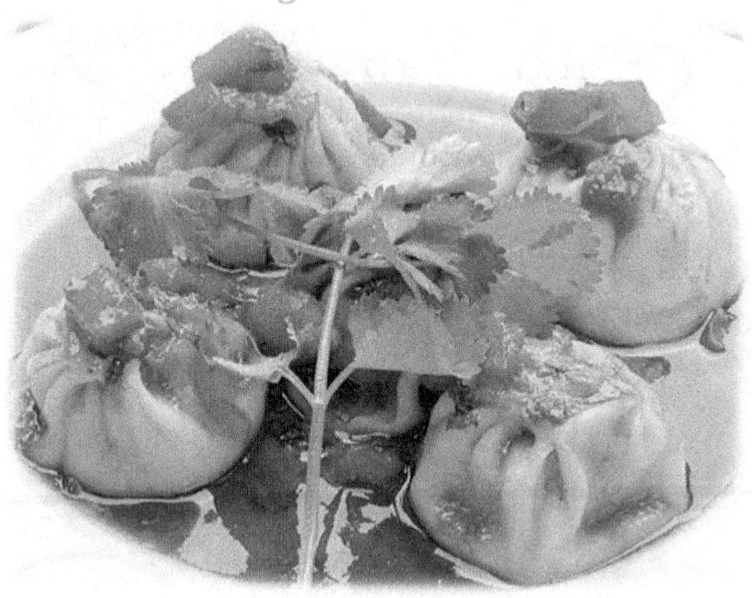

Ingredients:

- 2 finely chopped large onions
- 2 finely chopped bell peppers
- 8 carrots, finely chopped
- 200 g thinly shredded cabbage
- 2 jalapeno paprika
- 2 teaspoons garlic powder
- Some chopped coriander
- 200 g of mixed sprouts (soy, alfalfa)
- 2 tablespoons coconut aminos
- 1 teaspoon pepper
- 1 teaspoon salt for the filling + 1/2 teaspoon for the dough
- 200 g chickpea flour
- 4 tablespoons olive oil
- Some water for the dough

Directions:

1. Heat some oil in a sauce pan and sauté the onions along with bell peppers, carrots, shredded cabbage and sprouts for about 5-6 minutes.
2. Add some salt, chopped jalapeno chili, soy sauce, pepper, and toss well. Set aside.
3. Knead slightly firm dough using some chickpea flour, salt and water.
4. Roll the dough. Shape it into small circles.
5. Fill in the momo mixture one by one into these rolls and fold them gently.
6. Place the momos in a steamer and cook for about 12-15 minutes.
7. Serve them along with coconut aminos.

Nutritional Information per Serving:

Calories: 135; Total Fat: 2g; Carbs: 25.4g; Protein: 3.5g

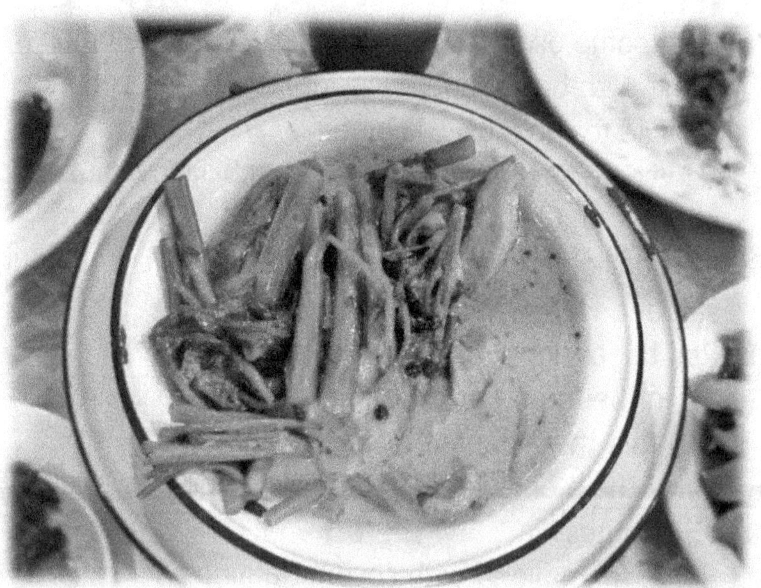

Ingredients:

- 120 g mustard leaves
- 400 g spinach, blanched
- 2 chopped green chili
- 6 minced garlic cloves
- 2 teaspoon minced ginger
- 1/2 teaspoon turmeric powder
- 4 finely chopped onions
- 4 chopped tomatoes
- 6 tablespoon chickpea flour
- 500 ml water
- 3 tablespoons of coconut oil
- Mustard seeds (3 tsp.)
- 1 teaspoon cumin
- 1 teaspoon salt
- 2 teaspoons maple syrup

Directions:

1. Take some water in a saucepan and throw in the mustard leaves, blanched spinach, ginger, chopped chili and cook it on a low flame for 20 minutes.
2. Once all the green veggies are cooked, blend them in a food processor until smooth.
3. Heat some coconut oil in another sauce pan. Next, add cumin then mustard seeds and let it crackle followed by turmeric powder.
4. Add the tomatoes and onions then sauté them for about 7-8 minutes.
5. Add green veggie paste to the saucepan and allow to cook for about 5 minutes.
6. Lastly add the chickpea flour, salt, maple syrup and cook for a few more minutes while continuously stirring the mixture.
7. Serve with gluten-free bread.

Nutritional Information per Serving:

Calories: 233.4; Total Fat: 8g; Carbs: 9.6g; Protein: 30g

Chapter Five: Salad Alkaline Diet Recipes

Spaghetti Mushroom Salad

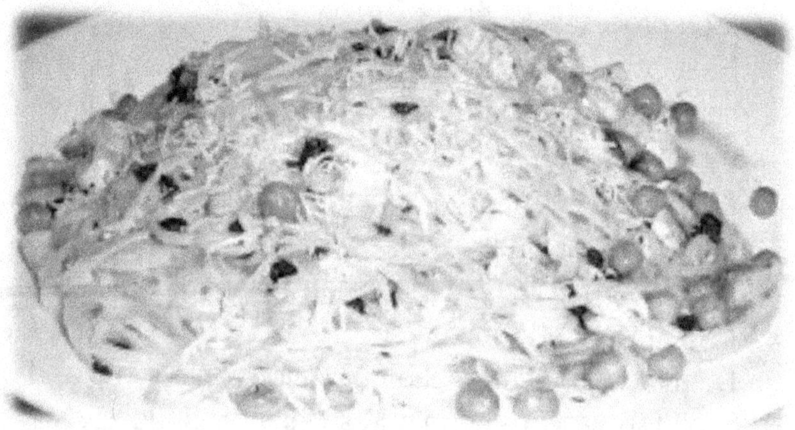

Ingredients:

- 300 g whole-wheat spaghetti
- 2 tablespoon sesame oil
- 2 minced garlic cloves
- 1 teaspoon minced ginger
- 2 teaspoon caraway seeds
- 60 g oyster mushrooms
- 100 g chopped kale leaves
- 2 tablespoons olive oil
- 2 chopped jalapeno pepper
- 2 tablespoons lemon juice
- Some chopped coriander
- 2 teaspoons salt
- 1 teaspoon pepper

Directions:

1. Boil some water in a large vessel, throw in the spaghetti and cook for about 7-8 minutes. Drain the water and set aside.
2. In another sauce pan, take some olive oil, sauté the minced garlic, ginger, caraway seeds. This should take a few minutes.
3. Add the mushrooms, kale leaves, jalapeno chili, pepper, salt and stir fry for 3-4 minutes.
4. Once cooled down, transfer the mixture from the saucepan to a large bowl. Add the boiled noodles, sprinkle some lemon juice and toss well.
5. Garnish with some toasted sesame seeds and serve.
6. Enjoy!

Nutritional Information per Serving:

Calories: 362.5; Total Fat: 13.8g; Carbs: 47.1g; Protein: 16.2g

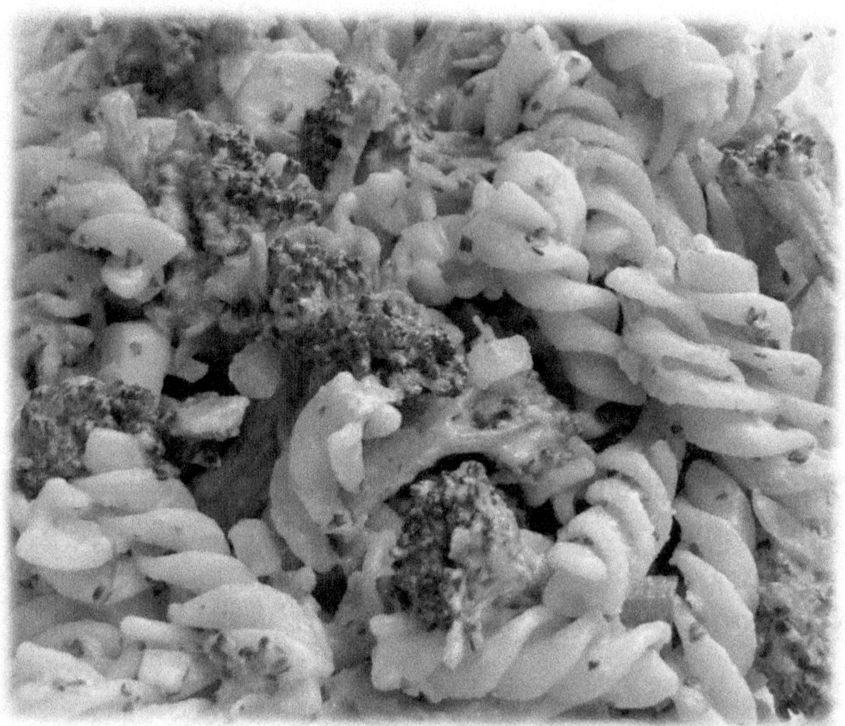

Ingredients:

- 150 g shitake or button mushrooms, chopped
- A handful of chopped and blanched kale leaves
- 160 g blanched broccoli florets
- 2 medium onion, sliced
- 4 tablespoons of olive oil
- 2 teaspoons pepper
- 1 teaspoon salt
- 100 g sprouts
- 2 teaspoons dark soy sauce
- 240 g soba noodles
- 1000 ml water to boil the noodles
- Some chopped parsley for garnish

Directions:

1. Take some water in a large sauce pan and bring it to a boil. Add half a teaspoon of olive oil so the noodles don't stick to each other.
2. Slide in the noodles and cook for about 3-4 minutes until they become slightly tender. Remember not to overcook the noodles. Drain the water. Set aside.
3. Take a salad bowl and mix the mushrooms along with kale leaves, broccoli florets, onion, noodles, pepper, salt, soy sauce and sprouts.
4. Drizzle some olive oil on top and toss.
5. Garnish with chopped parsley. Enjoy!

Nutritional Information per Serving:

Calories: 187.7; Total Fat: 11.1g; Carbs: 21.5g; Protein: 3.3g

Tomato Avocado Cucumber Salad

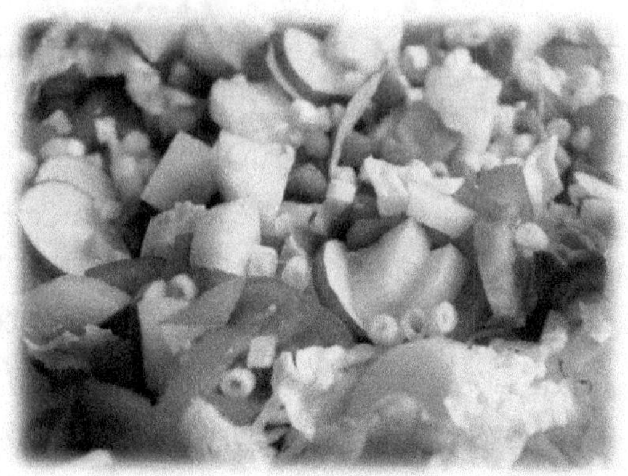

Ingredients:

- 2 avocados, peeled, pitted and sliced
- 4 big tomatoes
- 4 garlic cloves, minced
- 150 g arugula leaves
- 40 g cilantro
- 2 cucumbers, peeled and sliced
- 1 apple, peeled and sliced
- 200 g of basmati rice, cooked and cooled
- 60 g almonds
- A pinch of salt
- Juice of 2 lemons
- 120 ml coconut milk
- 1 teaspoon curry powder

Directions:

1. Place all the salad ingredients in a bowl and stir well.
2. Mix lemon juice with coconut oil, Himalayan salt and curry powder.
3. Spread the salsa over the salad.
4. Enjoy!

Nutritional Information per Serving:

Calories: 90.2; Total Fat: 4.6g; Carbs: 10.7g; Protein: 3.3g

Spinach Bean Tomato Salad

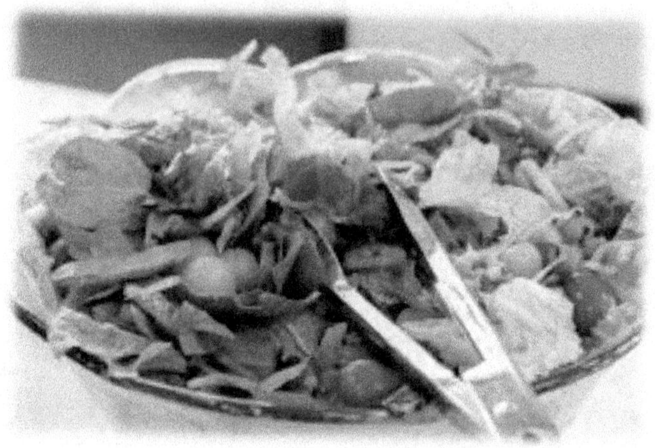

Ingredients:

- 200 g chickpea, soaked overnight
- 160 g black beans, soaked overnight
- 4 cucumbers, peeled and chopped
- 2 medium onions, finely chopped
- 2 chopped tomatoes
- 2 chopped raw mangos
- 15 spinach leaves
- 2 teaspoons ground cumin
- 2 teaspoons raw mango powder
- 1 teaspoon salt
- 1 teaspoon cayenne pepper
- Some chopped cilantro
- 2x 1000 ml water to boil the beans and chickpeas

Directions:

1. Boil the chickpeas and black beans in water. Drain and set aside.
2. Boil some additional water in another vessel and blanch the spinach for about 30 seconds. Drain the water.

3. In a large bowl, combine the chickpeas, blanched lettuce, cumin, onion, chopped raw mango, dry mango powder, pepper, tomato, salt and mix well.
4. Garnish with some chopped cilantro and serve.
5. Enjoy!

Nutritional Information per Serving:

Calories: 319.7; Total Fat: 22.8g; Carbs: 22.4g; Protein: 11.8g

Jalapeno Pomegranate Salad

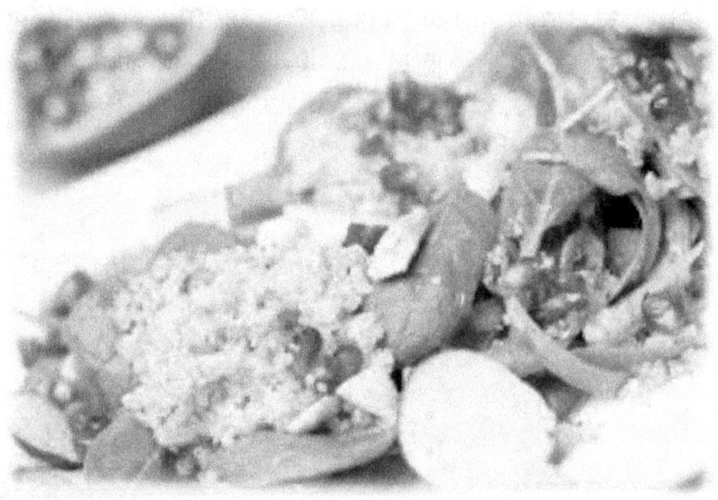

Ingredients:

- 240 g chopped apples
- 300 g cucumber, peeled and sliced
- 300 g pomegranate seeds
- 2 Jalapeño Peppers
- 2 medium onions, peeled and chopped
- 25 raw almonds
- 2 minced garlic cloves
- 2 tablespoons lemon juice
- 1 teaspoon lemon zest
- A teaspoon of pepper powder
- 4 tablespoons raisins
- 16 lettuce leaves
- 1 teaspoon salt
- 2 tablespoons olive oil
- A handful of wakame seaweed, previously soaked in water as per instructions

Directions:

1. Combine all the ingredients in a big bowl, starting with all the veggies, then the fruits, wakame and spices.
2. Drizzle some olive oil on top and toss well. Add salt to taste.
3. Serve immediately or refrigerate for 2 hours.

Nutritional Information per Serving:

Calories: 83.5; Total Fat: 3.9g; Carbs: 12.1g; Protein: 1.9g

Chapter Six: Snacks Alkaline Diet Recipes

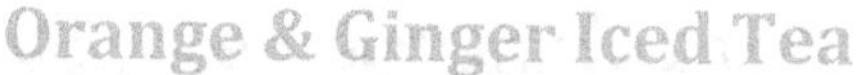

Orange & Ginger Iced Tea

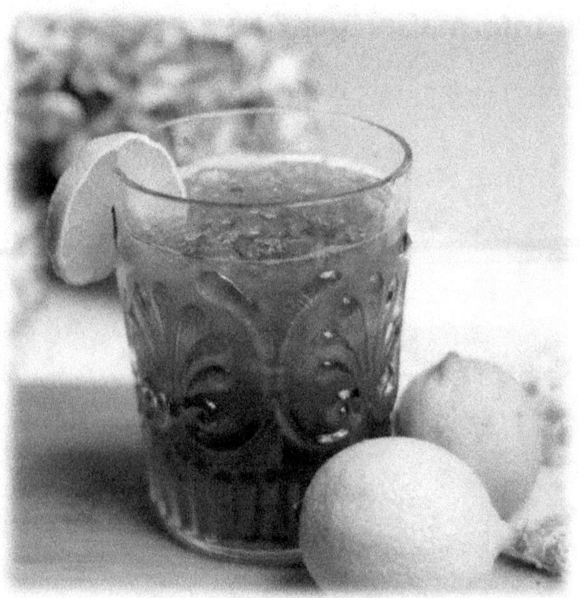

Ingredients

- 2 inches fresh ginger, cut into slices
- 1 medium orange
- 4 cups filtered water
- 1 cup cold filtered water

Directions

1. Place the ginger slices into a saucepan with the 4 cups of filtered water. Bring to the boil, then simmer for 10 minutes.

2. Next grate the zest from the orange and squeeze the juice (in that order) and add to the ginger and water mixture.
3. Strain the mixture and leave until completely cool.
4. Add the iced water and place in the fridge until you're ready to enjoy it.

Nutritional Information per Serving:

Calories: 77; Total Fat: 0g; Carbs: 19g; Protein: 1g

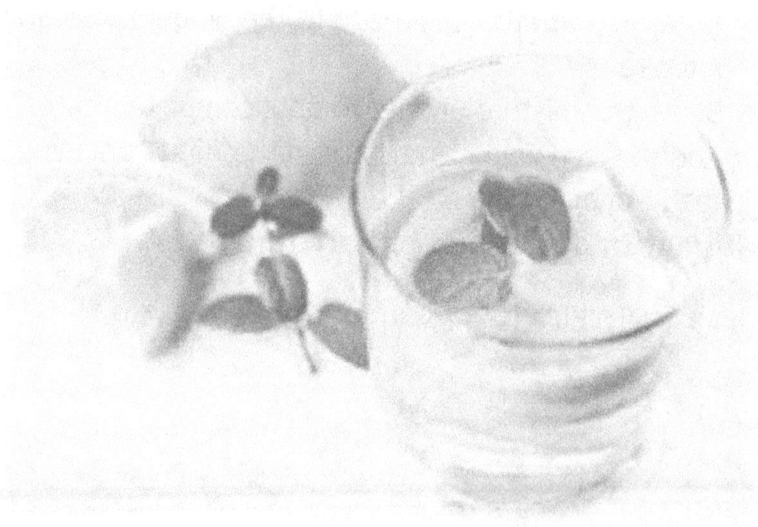

Ingredients:

- 1-gallon filtered water
- 1 cucumber
- 0.5 grapefruit
- 1 lemon
- 6 mint leaves

Directions:

1. Pour the water into a glass container that allows for at least three inches of additional space.
2. Slice your fruit and cucumber.
3. Place the fruit, mint, and cucumber into the water.
4. Allow it to chill overnight. Enjoy.

Nutritional Information per Serving:

Calories: 1.3; Total Fat: 0g; Carbs: 0.4g; Protein: 0g

Mojito Water

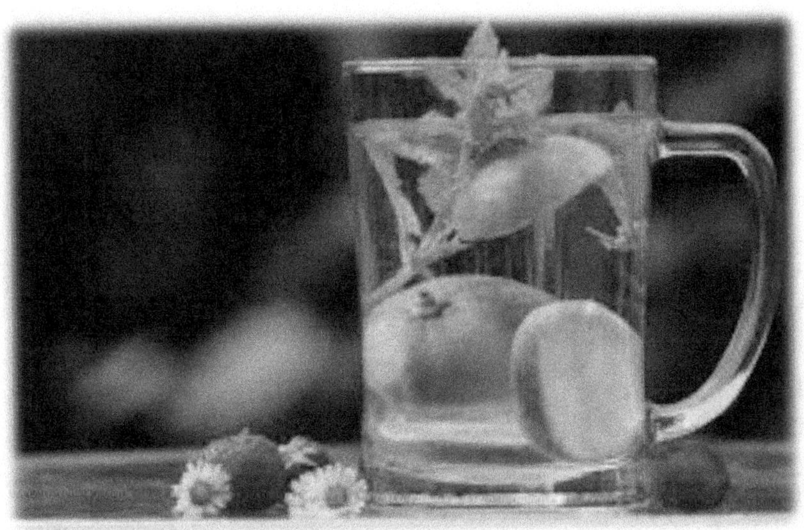

Ingredients:

- 1-gallon filtered water
- 2 limes
- 6 mint leaves
- 1 lemon
- 1 cucumber

Directions:

1. Put the water into a glass container that leaves room for the other Ingredients.
2. Cut up your fruit and cucumber.
3. Place the ingredients into the water.
4. Allow it chill overnight.

Nutritional Information per Serving:

Calories: 0; Total Fat: 0g; Carbs: 0g; Protein: 0g

Perfect Peach & Mint Iced Tea

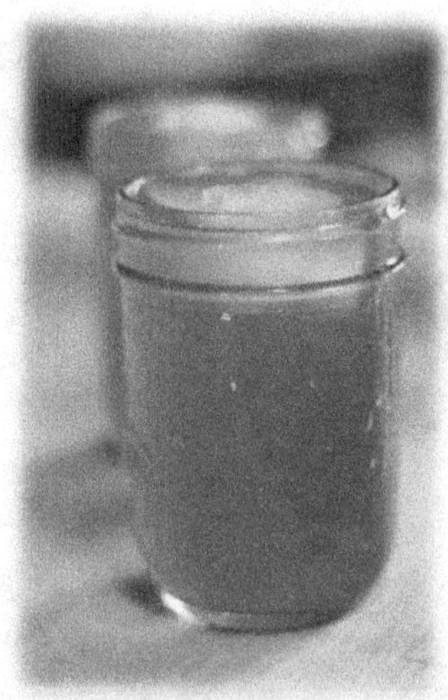

Ingredients:

- 4 large peaches
- 1 tablespoon fresh or dried mint leaves
- 4 cups filtered water
- Juice of ½ lemon

Directions:

1. Firstly, place mint leaves or mint tea bag into a bowl, cover with boiling water and leave for 5-10 minutes for the flavor to infuse. Leave until completely cooled.
2. De-stone and peel the peaches and blend with a small amount of water until smooth.
3. Combine the cooled tea with the peach puree and add lemon juice, pour into a mason jar and then place in the fridge.
4. Drink and enjoy!

Nutritional Information per Serving:

Calories: 32; Total Fat: 0g; Carbs: 32g; Protein: 1g

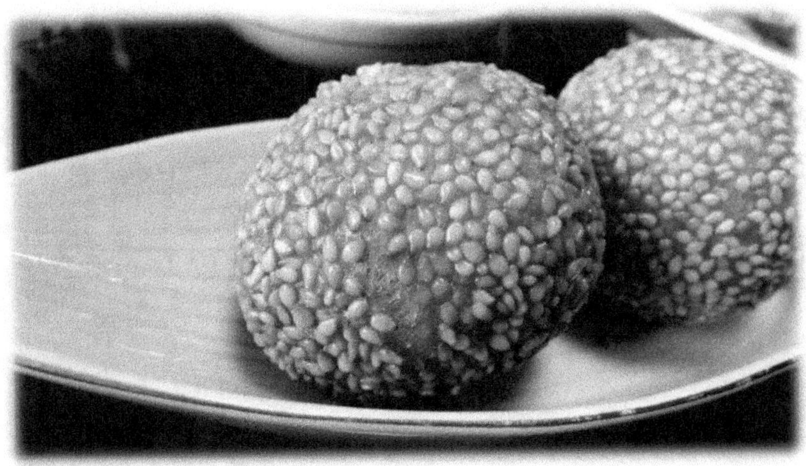

Ingredients:

- 1 cup almond butter, raw
- 0.25 cups flax seeds
- 3 teaspoons chia seeds
- 0.25 cups chia seeds (additional)
- 3 teaspoons cinnamon
- 1 cup hemp seeds, hulled
- 6 dates that do not contain any pits
- 0.25 cups cacao nibs
- 2 teaspoons vanilla

Directions:

1. Process the dates and almond butter.
2. Add all the ingredients, except the 3-teaspoon portion of the hemp seeds.
3. Process all the ingredients well.
4. Place the dough on a board.
5. Roll into small balls.

6. Put the 3-teaspoon portions of hemp seeds into a small bowl.
7. Roll the ball in the seeds.
8. Place in a container that is completely airtight.
9. Enjoy for up to a week.

Nutritional Information per Serving:

Calories: 104.8; Total Fat: 3.6g; Carbs: 16g; Protein: 3.6g

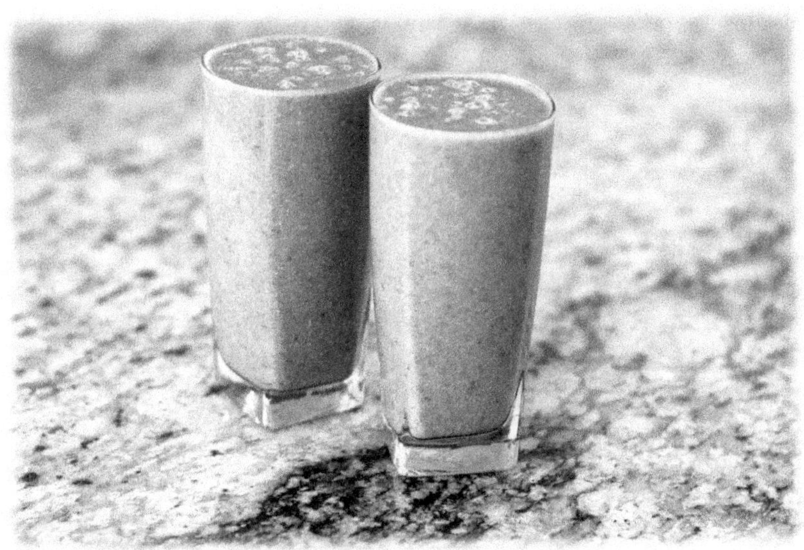

Ingredients:

- 1 cup coconut water
- 0.5 banana
- Dash of cinnamon
- 1 tablespoon chia seeds
- 1 handful spinach
- 1 pear
- 1 tablespoon coconut oil

Directions:

1. Place all ingredients in a blender.
2. Process until fully smooth.

Nutritional Information per Serving:

Calories: 171.2; Total Fat: 0.8g; Carbs: 37g; Protein: 4g

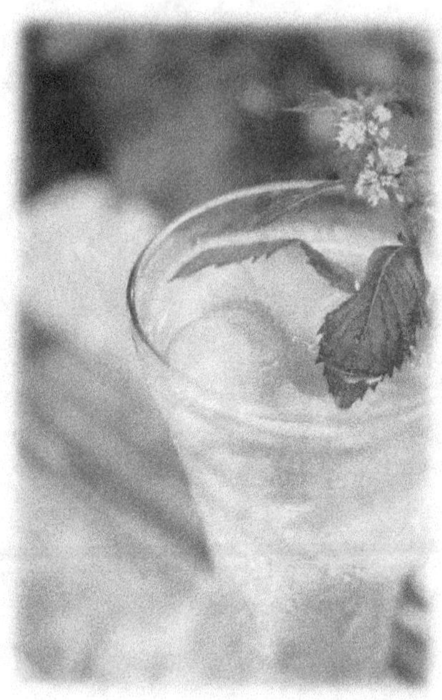

Ingredients:

- 8 cups filtered water
- 3 mint leaves
- 2 cups watermelon

Directions:

1. Pour the water into a glass container.
2. Chop the watermelon.
3. Put in the mint and watermelon.
4. Allow it to sit overnight.

Nutritional Information per Serving:

Calories: 47; Total Fat: 0.6g; Carbs: 11.6g; Protein: 1g

Cranberry Smoothie

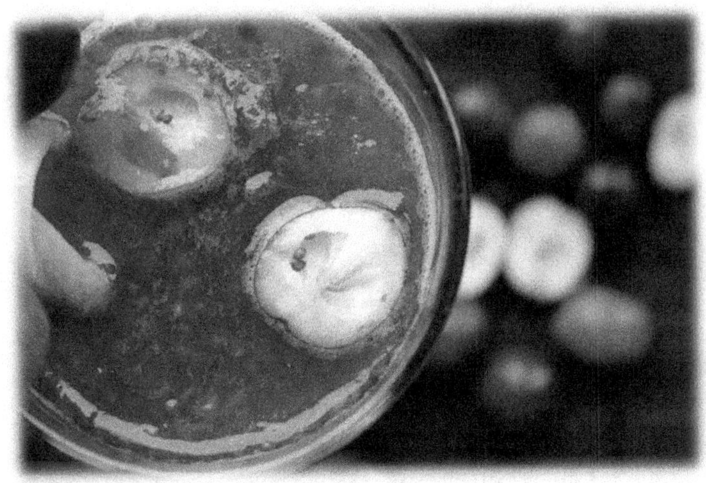

Ingredients:

- 2 cups coconut water
- 1 cup cranberries
- 1 avocado
- 2 teaspoons ginger
- 0.025 teaspoons cinnamon
- 0.5 cups almonds
- 1 cup spinach
- 2 tablespoons lemon juice
- 1 date
- 0.5 cups ice

Directions:

1. Place all ingredients in a blender.
2. Process until fully smooth.

Nutritional Information per Serving:

Calories: 324; Total Fat: 10g; Carbs: 59g; Protein: 8g

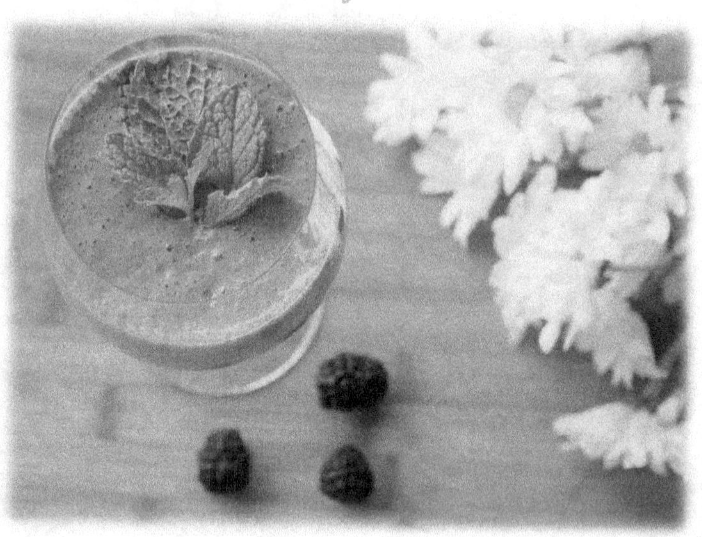

Ingredients:

- 1.5 cups coconut milk
- 1 kale bunch
- 2 tablespoons coconut oil
- 1 cup blackberries
- 1 lime
- 0.5 cups strawberries
- 0.5 teaspoons vanilla

Directions:

1. Blend the milk and kale.
2. Squeeze the lime juice into the blender.
3. Add the remaining ingredients individually.
4. Blend until it's smooth.

Nutritional Information per Serving:

Calories: 249; Total Fat: 1.5g; Carbs: 60.5g; Protein: 6.3g

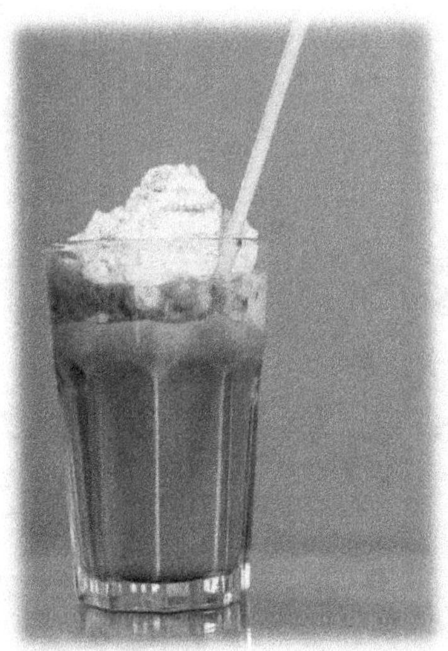

Ingredients:

- 0.25 cups raw almonds
- 1 cup coconut milk
- 0.5 cups mint leaves
- 1 teaspoon chia seeds
- 4 pitted dates
- 2 tablespoons cacao nibs
- 0.5 avocado
- 1 cup ice

Directions:

1. Place all ingredients in a blender.
2. Process until fully smooth.

Nutritional Information per Serving:

Calories: 306; Total Fat: 7.4g; Carbs: 43.2g; Protein: 19.2g

Chapter Seven: Deserts Alkaline Diet Recipes

Spiced Melon and Fig Smoothie

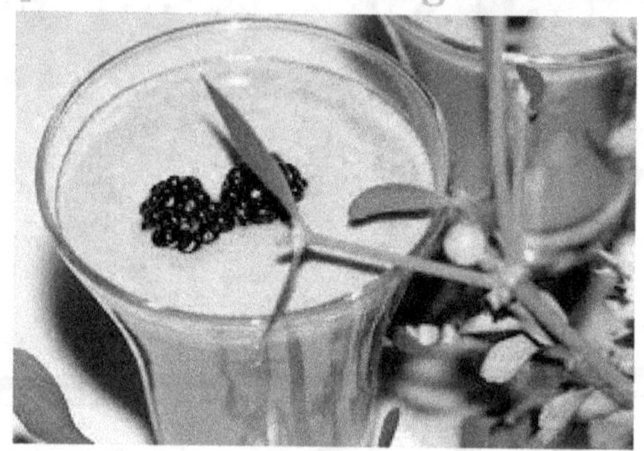

Ingredients:

- 2 cups cantaloupe, cubed
- 3 figs, fresh
- 3 cups fresh baby spinach
- 1 medium mango
- ½ teaspoon ground cinnamon

Directions:

1. First place the melon in your blender and blend until smooth. Then add the spinach and blend again.
2. Next peel and de-stone the mango.
3. Add the mango to the blender along with the rest of the ingredients and blend until smooth and creamy. Enjoy!

Nutritional Information per Serving:

Calories: 113.5; Total Fat: 1.7g; Carbs: 22.1g; Protein: 4.3g

Beetroot Almond Pudding

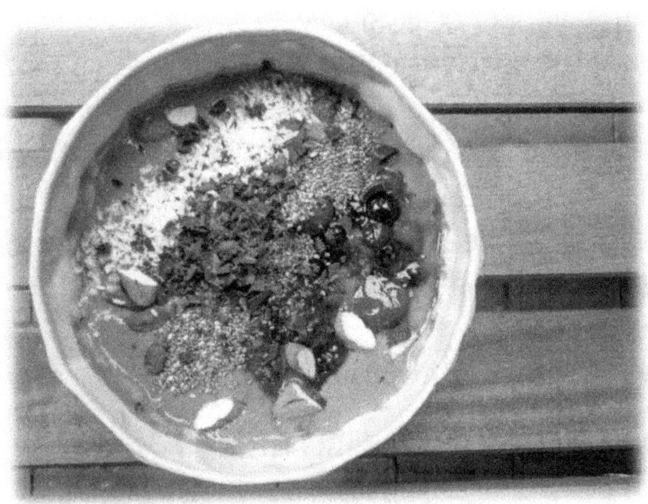

Ingredients:

- 600 g peeled and shredded beetroot
- 2 tablespoons coconut oil
- 4 tablespoons of almond butter
- 500 ml almond milk
- 2 teaspoons cardamom powder
- 1/2 teaspoon nutmeg powder
- 15chopped almonds
- 15 chopped cashews
- 80 g raisins

Directions:

1. Heat the coconut oil in a large sauce pan. Cook the shredded beetroot for about 12-15 minutes on low heat with the lid covered. Give it an occasional stir.
2. Add cardamom powder, almond milk and butter, nutmeg powder, raisins and cook for another 10-12

minutes on low heat. Remember to cover the saucepan with a lid. Stir occasionally.

3. Once the mixture cools down, refrigerate it for 60-90 minutes.
4. Heat another sauce pan and slightly roast the chopped almonds and cashews.
5. Garnish the beetroot pudding with toasted almonds and cashews on top.
6. Serve chilled.

Nutritional Information per Serving:

Calories: 94.7; Total Fat: 0.7g; Carbs: 23.6g; Protein: 3g

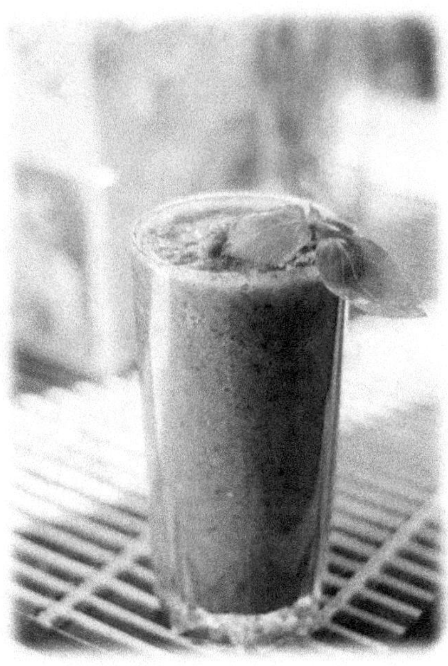

Ingredients

- 1 cup frozen cherries
- Juice of 1 lime
- 1 cup (250ml) coconut water
- Generous handful of basil leaves

Directions:

1. Pour coconut water into your blender, add basil and blend until smooth.
2. Add to this the cherries and lime juice.
3. Blend until smooth and enjoy!

Nutritional Information per Serving:

Calories: 138; Total Fat: 0g; Carbs: 30g; Protein: 0g

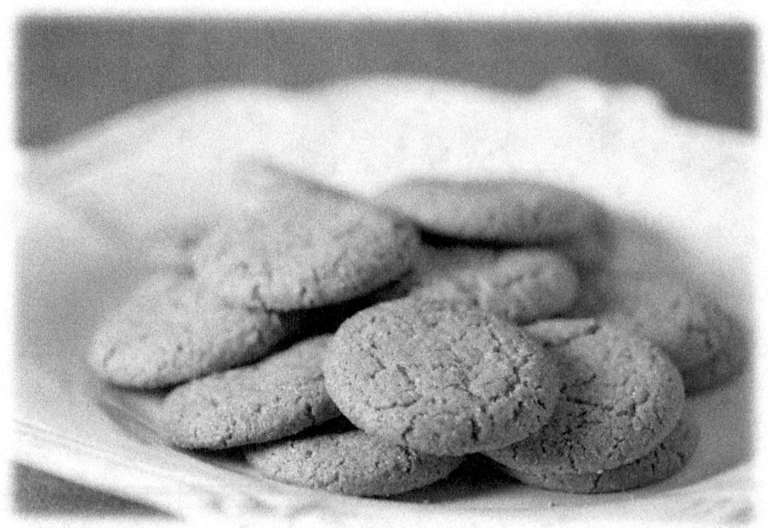

Ingredients:

- 200 g coarsely ground almond flour
- 80 g gluten-free oats
- 60 g coconut flour
- 2 tsp. baking powder
- 2 tbsp. cinnamon powder
- 2 tbsp. ginger powder
- 1 teaspoon all-spice powder
- 1 teaspoon nutmeg powder
- 2 teaspoons vanilla essence
- 14 tablespoons coconut oil
- 120 ml almond milk for binding

Directions:

1. In a large bowl, combine almond flour, coconut flour, oats, baking powder, cinnamon, all spice powder, ginger, nutmeg powder and mix well.
2. Add vanilla essence, coconut oil, almond milk.

3. Set this mixture in the refrigerator for about 25-30 minutes until it becomes slightly firm.
4. Preheat the oven to 350°F/180°C.
5. Split the cookie dough into 18-20 circular balls and place them on a baking sheet.
6. Bake the cookies for about 15 mins. Let them cool down.
7. Transfer them into an air-tight container and enjoy the cookies during breakfast or as an evening snack.
8. Enjoy!

Nutritional Information per Serving:

Calories: 119.8; Total Fat: 6.1g; Carbs: 13.6g; Protein: 1.7g

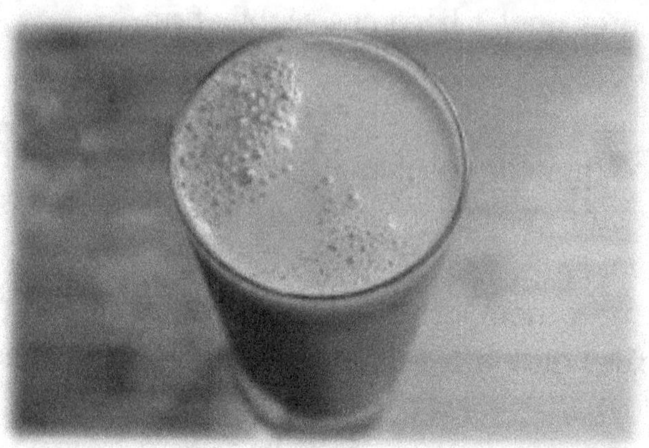

Ingredients:

- 1 ripe peach
- 1 ripe banana
- 6 kale leaves (without spines)
- 1 cup (250ml) coconut water

Directions:

1. Pour the coconut water into your blender. Add the kale and blend until smooth.
   Next peel the banana and de-stone the peach.
2. In your blender, add the fruit to the spinach-coconut water mixture and blitz until smooth.
3. Enjoy!

Nutritional Information per Serving:

Calories: 155.5; Total Fat: 0.3g; Carbs: 30.2g; Protein: 11g

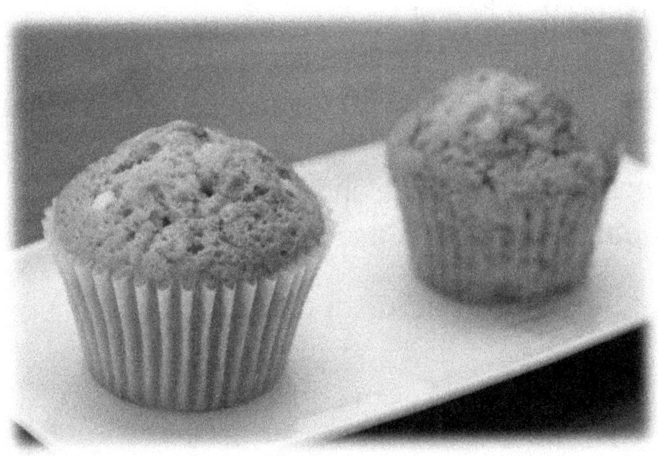

Ingredients:

- 340 g quinoa, cooked and dried
- 140 g whole-wheat flour
- 2 teaspoons baking powder
- 1 teaspoon baking soda
- 2 tablespoons toasted flax seeds
- 4 ripe bananas, mashed
- 4 teaspoons vanilla essence
- 2 sweet potatoes, boiled and mashed
- 240 g applesauce, unsweetened
- 1 teaspoon cinnamon
- 1 teaspoon salt

Directions:

1. Preheat the oven to 390°F/200°C.
2. In a bowl, combine the quinoa along with salt, flax seeds, baking powder, baking soda, and flour.
3. In another bowl, combine all the wet ingredients like applesauce, banana and mashed sweet potato.

4. Transfer the wet ingredients to the dry ones and mix well using a beater.
5. Pour this batter into each muffin tin one by one.
6. Bake them for about 50 minutes to get fluffy and moist muffins.
7. Cool down in a fridge and enjoy!

Nutritional Information per Serving:

Calories: 146.5; Total Fat: 6.1g; Carbs: 50.1g; Protein: 3.3g

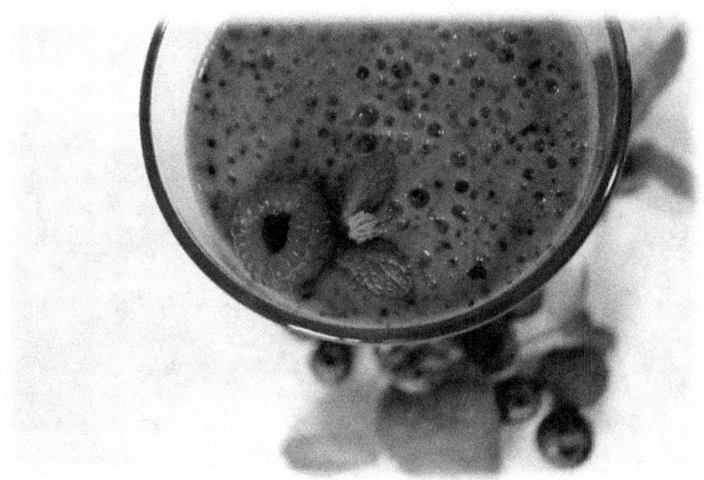

Ingredients

- 1 ripe banana (or more if hungry)
- 1 cup (140g approx.) blackberries, raspberries or strawberries, fresh or frozen
- Handful fresh baby spinach
- Juice of ½ lemon

Directions:

1. Blend the baby spinach leaves in a small amount of water.
2. Peel your banana and add to the spinach in your blender, and also the rest of the ingredients.
3. Blend until smooth and creamy.
4. Enjoy!

Nutritional Information per Serving:

Calories: 210; Total Fat: 0g; Carbs: 55g; Protein: 0g

Peach Almond Chia Smoothie

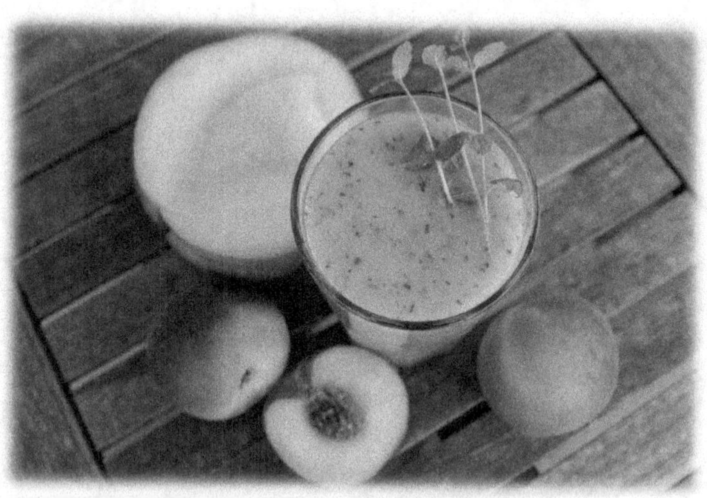

Ingredients:

- 5 ripe peaches, diced
- 1 teaspoon cardamom powder
- 1 banana, chopped
- 120 ml lemon juice
- 1000 ml almond milk
- 2 teaspoons chia seeds
- Some ice cubes

Directions:

1. Combine the diced peaches, banana, almond milk and orange juice in a food processor and blend until smooth.
2. Sprinkle some cardamom powder and stir it well.
3. Pour the smoothie into large glasses.
4. Add some ice cubes and enjoy!

Nutritional Information per Serving:

Calories: 331; Total Fat: 0.7g; Carbs: 59g; Protein: 11g

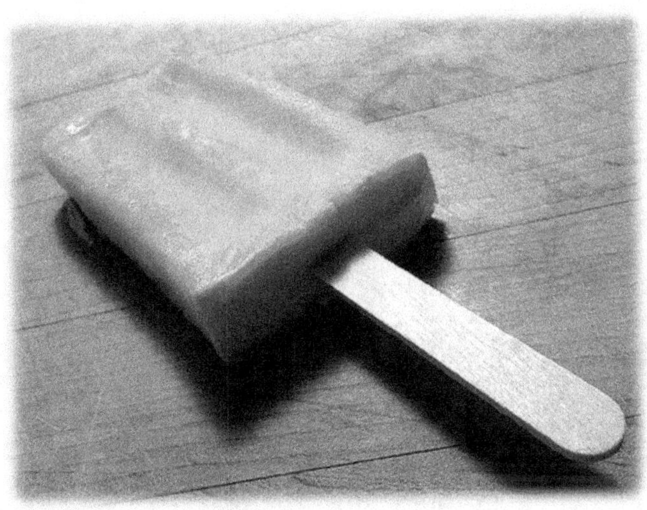

Ingredients:

- 4 fresh carrots, ends trimmed
- 1 raw medium sweet potato, peeled
- 2 medium oranges
- 1 lime

Directions:

1. Peel the oranges, lime and sweet potato. Top and tail the carrots.
2. Add all of the ingredients to your juicer.
3. Juice (strain if necessary) and enjoy!

Nutritional Information per Serving:

Calories: 450; Total Fat: 2g; Carbs: 102g; Protein: 3g

Coconut Pumpkin Smoothie

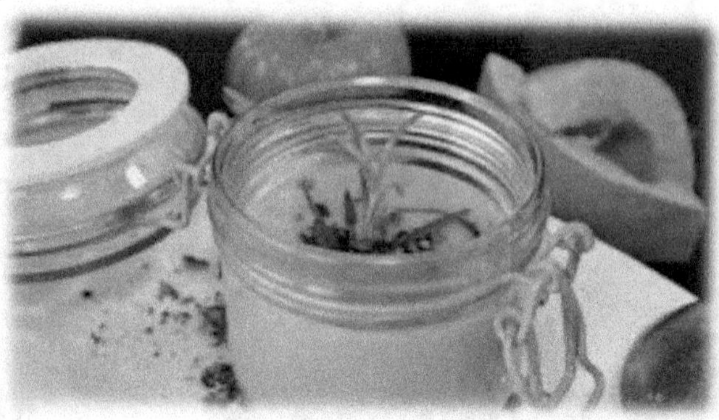

Ingredients:

- 300 g chopped pumpkin, steamed
- 500 ml coconut milk
- 120 ml almond milk
- 1 avocado
- 1/2 teaspoon cinnamon powder
- 1/2 teaspoon all-spice powder
- 1/2 teaspoon nutmeg powder
- 2 teaspoons vanilla essence
- 2 tablespoons flax seeds
- A few drops of stevia
- Some ice cubes

Directions:

1. Blend until smooth.
2. Pour this pumpkin smoothie into a large glass.
3. Add some ice cubes and serve. Enjoy!

Nutritional Information per Serving:

Calories: 263.7; Total Fat: 5.5g; Carbs: 28.2g; Protein: 27.6g

Conclusion

Thank you so much for sticking with us to the end of The Alkaline Diet Guide for Beginners! I hope you have enjoyed all the information we had to share and cooking all 50 Alkaline Diet recipes with us.

The next step is to continue mixing and matching as you enjoy great food and healthier life. Be sure to join us again on another one of our other amazing culinary adventures, and if you enjoyed my work, go ahead and leave a positive review on my Amazon page!

Until then, keep cooking, and moving towards all your culinary goals. All the best!

DEAR READER,
THANK YOU FOR BUYING AND READING MY BOOK!
IF YOU LIKE IT, PLEASE, LEAVE A REVIEW. IT IS
IMPORTANT FOR ME AND MY FUTURE BOOKS.
JUST SCAN THIS QR CODE AND YOU CAN LEAVE A
REVIEW

OR JUST TYPE THIS LINK–

HTTPS://WWW.AMAZON.COM/REVIEW/CREATE-REVIEW?IE=UTF8&ASIN=B07C7GD9CF#